The Great Lover
Playbook

The Great Lover

Playbook

(formerly *365 Days of Sensational Sex*)

365 Sexual Tips and Techniques to
Keep the Fires Burning All Year Long

Lou Paget

Anchor Canada

Library and Archives Canada Cataloguing in Publication data has been applied for.

Text illustrations by Diego Felipe
Designed by Sabrina Bowers
Printed and bound in the USA

Published in Canada by
Anchor Canada, a division of
Random House of Canada Limited

Visit Random House of Canada Limited's website: www.randomhouse.ca

BVG   10   9   8   7   6   5   4   3   2

To my sisters
Diane Paget-Dellio (the Raptor),
Sherry Paget (the Wiz),
and Kathie Ireland (Katerena),
with all my love

&

To all who have shared their lives,
their loves, their experiences,
and to all who asked for this book

Contents

Acknowledgments   xix
Introduction   xxi

How to Be a Great Lover in Attitude

1. Falling-in-Love Sex vs. Being-in-Love Sex.   1
2. Sex Beyond Intercourse.   2
3. Give Yourselves Permission.   3
4. Know There Is Always More to Know about Sex.   4
5. Treat Her Like a Lady.   4
6. Gentlemen, Let Her Know You Want to Make Her Come—
   Anytime, Anywhere, Anyhow.   5
7. Ladies, Remember That Oral Sex Isn't Just for Dating.   6
8. Let Him Be the Man.   7
9. Stay Current.   8
10. Vulnerability = Value.   8
11. The Legacy of Trusting.   9
12. Relationship As Refuge.   9
13. Intellectual Freedom.   10
14. Cherish.   11
15. Love vs. Lust.   11

16. Stand Up for Your Rights.   12
17. Sowing Roots.   13
18. Frequency Is Dynamic.   13
19. A Calm before the Storm.   14
20. Relish How Your Body Makes Your Lover Feel.   14
21. Are You Willing to Talk Dirty?   15
22. Are You Open to Enhancers?   15
23. Great Lover Moment: Great Lovers Are Shrewd Consumers.   16
24. Be Brave Enough to Share Your Innermost Fantasies.   17
25. Be Willing to Change Something about Your Appearance
    to Suit Your Lover's Preference.   18
26. Be Willing to Listen to Your Lover's Complaints about You.   18
27. Be Gentle When Airing a Disappointment or Hurt
    Caused by Your Partner.   19
28. Practice Approaching Your Partner from a Point of View
    of Mutual Respect, Not Blame or Defensiveness.   19
29. The Gift of Giving.   20
30. The Richness of Receiving.   20
31. Great Sex Is Chronologically Ageless.   21
32. Great Lover Moment: "I Still Completely Dig Her."   22
33. The Crying Connection.   22
34. Touch Your Lover's Heart and Soul.   23
35. Insisting on Being Right Can Kill Your Sex Life and Threaten
    Your Relationship.   24
36. Be Proud of Each Other.   25
37. Never Think of Love As Work.   26
38. Remember That the Way You Treat Him or Her at 8 A.M.
    Impacts the Way He or She Treats You at 8 P.M.   26
39. Protect What Is Yours.   27
40. Health Benefits of Frequent Sex.   28
41. Great Lover Moment: "She Rejuvenates Me."   28
42. Lust's Triumvirate.   29
43. Build a Stone House.   29
44. Accept That Some Problems Can't Be Solved.   30
45. Beyond Orgasms.   31
46. Always Be a Beginner.   32
47. Live in a Culture of Appreciation.   32
48. Nurture Those Values You Have in Common.   34
49. Nurture Those Values Related to Family.   34
50. Nurture Those Values Related to Your Spiritual Life.   35
51. Nurture Those Values Related to Work.   36
52. Nurture Those Values Related to Money.   37
53. Court Your Lover, Forever.   38

54. Je Ne Sais Quoi—or "I Just Can't Explain It."   39
55. Seasonal Sex.   40
56. Timetables Are for Trains.   40
57. Enlarge Your Expectations—for Yourself, Your Lover,
    and Your Relationship.   41
58. Minimize Your Expectations—for Yourself, Your Lover,
    and Your Relationship.   42
59. Let Passion and Sex Be a Reward for You As a Couple,
    Not a Chore or Obligation.   43
60. Don't Get Carried Away by Performance.   43
61. Make Lovemaking a Conscious Lifestyle Choice.   44
62. You Are Committed 24/7.   44
63. Style Differences.   45
64. Be Honest and Forgiving of Your Own Human Frailties.   45
65. Be Honest and Forgiving of Your Lover's Human Frailties.   46
66. Understand That All Aspects of Your Relationship Affect Your
    Sexual Relationship.   46
67. Understand That Separating the Various Aspects of Your
    Relationship Can Put Those Parts at Risk.   47
68. Be Open to "Tune-Ups."   47
69. Be Willing to Challenge Your Own Sexual Comfort Zone.   48
70. Remember That Just Because It Isn't Important to You
    Doesn't Mean It Isn't Important to Her.   49

How to Be a Great Lover in Behavior

71. Speak to Each Other As You Did When You First Met.   51
72. Gentlemen, Let Her Know She's Irresistible.   52
73. Ladies, Let Him Know He's Irresistible.   53
74. Great Lover Moment: "I Simply Can't Get Enough of Her."   53
75. Take the Pulse of a Relationship on an Ongoing Basis.   53
76. Ladies, Acknowledge the Things He Does for You.   55
77. Gentlemen, Pay Deep Attention to Her—in Whatever Way
    She Wants.   55
78. Act Quickly to Spot and Fix a Problem.   58
79. Learn from Your Mistakes.   59
80. Be an Explorer.   60
81. No Psychic Sex.   61
82. Seal Your Lips.   62
83. Don't Compare Yourselves to Anyone, Much Less Hollywood Idols.   63
84. Live by Your Own Script, Dance to Your Own Drummer,
    and Sing Your Own Song.   64

85. Romancing the Stone.   64
86. Never Embarrass Each Other.   65
87. Maintain Your Dignity.   66
88. Diplomatic Corps in the Bedroom.   66
89. Keep Talking.   67
90. Learn How to Compromise.   67
91. Be Tastefully Jealous—Possess Your Lover Culturally and Socially.   68
92. Don't Push Your Lover's Buttons.   69
93. Arguing Is Not Always a Bad Thing.   70
94. Fight Fair (or Learn How To).   71
95. Are You Clean Enough?   73
96. Ask and You Shall Receive.   74
97. Be Patient in Creating Your Relationship Even Though Being
     Patient May Not Be Your Strongest Virtue.   74
98. Great Lover Moment: Take Your Time.   74
99. Don't Be Susceptible to Instant Gratification.   75
100. Money Is the Third Dynamic of a Relationship.   76
101. Treat Your Relationship Like It Is a Living Thing.   76
102. Support and Respect Each Other's Personal Endeavors.   77
103. Give Each Other Space.   78
104. Fight for Your Relationship in Times of Stress.   78
105. Listen to Your Little Voice.   79
106. Be a Great Toucher.   80
107. Turn Off the TV.   83
108. No Kids in the Bed!   83
109. Home Is Where the Heart Is.   84
110. Hug Each Other.   84
111. Create Emotional Safety.   85
112. Gentlemen, Remember That Your Fingers and Hands Are
     a Wonderful Source of Pleasure for Your Lady.   86
113. Turn Complaints into Requests.   86
114. Create Important Moments and Make Memories.   88
115. Make Your Lover Laugh.   89
116. Friends and Family Matter.   89
117. Allow Your Partner to Take Credit for Stories,
     without Correction or Editing.   90
118. Spend Time Alone.   91
119. Spend Time Alone, Together.   91
120. Dine Together Often.   92
121. Is Your Lover One of Your Top Priorities?   92
122. Reinvent Dinner.   92
123. Plan Trips.   93
124. Plan Outings.   94

125. Plan Sex! 94
126. Take Care of Your Body. 95
127. Encourage Your Lover to Take Care of His or Her Body. 96
128. Good Grooming. 96
129. Take Care of Your Emotional and Mental Health. 98
130. Remember to Speak Compliments Out Loud. 99
131. Gentlemen, Always Do What You Say You Are Going to Do. 99
132. Seek Out the Solace of Physical Contact. 100
133. Ladies, Go into His Physical Space and Hug Your Man. 100
134. Cuddle First Thing in the Morning. 101
135. Don't Go Looking for Trouble. 101
136. Buy Each Other Garments That Only the Two of You Will See. 102
137. Give Your Partner Downtime upon Returning Home after Work. 102
138. Don't Keep a Running List of Who Did What to Whom. 103
139. Take Pleasure in the Little Things. 103

Great Lover Tips and Techniques

140. Ladies, Know What Turns Him On. 106
141. Great Lover Moment: "My Dear, I Would Really Like a Slice
    of Pie Tonight." 106
142. Gentlemen, Know What Turns Her On. 107
143. Gentlemen, Know What Turns Her Off. 108
144. Gentlemen, Get Connected. 109
145. Gentlemen, Love Her Body. 110
146. Great Lover Moment: The Truth Is in the Photos. 110
147. Gentlemen, Stay Connected During the Day. 110
148. Ladies, Know What Turns Him Off. 111
149. What Are Your Three Hot Buttons? 111
150. Create Your Own Love-Life Response Sheet. 112
151. Show-and-Tell for Grown-Ups. 112
152. Linger in the Pleasures of Foreplay. 113
153. Window Dressing for Undressing—for Him. 113
154. Red Light, Green Light—for Her. 114
155. The Sock Drawer—for Him. 115
156. A Call That Says a Thousand Words—for Her. 115
157. Anatomy Lesson—for Her. 116
158. Playing with the Mannequin—for Him or Her. 116
159. Spectator Sports for Two. 116
160. Dance Together. 116
161. Flirt at a Party and Leave Early. 117
162. Learn How to Praise Specific Techniques. 117

163. Learn How to Critique Specific Techniques without Being Hurtful.   118
164. Fasting Leads to Sexual Feasting.   118
165. Garner Sexual Inspiration from Any Source.   118
166. Maintain the Heat of Intimacy Regardless of How Many Miles
Apart You May Be.   119
167. Make It a Point to Find out How Your Lover Likes to Be Kissed.   120
168. Never Stop Kissing.   121
169. Ladies, Use His Body for Your Sexual Pleasure, Again and Again.   122
170. Set the Scene in Your Brain, and Then Create the Opportunity.   122
171. Learn How to Transform a Quiet Evening in Front of the TV
into One That Is Not So Quiet.   123
172. Initiate Sex.   124
173. Make Any Venue a Place for a Sexual Encounter.   124
174. Ladies, Rather Than Rush to Clean up after Sex, Whet Your Man's
Primal Power and Leave Some of Him Inside of You.   125
175. Gentlemen, Move the Target on Her Pleasure.   126
176. Expand Your Sexual Library.   127
177. Don't Worry about Making a Mess.   127
178. Develop Different Styles of Lovemaking.   127
179. Hide-and-Seek Sex.   128
180. Silence Is Golden.   128
181. Blindfolded Sex.   129
182. The Pleasures of Comfort Sex.   129
183. Investigate Baby-Making Sex.   129
184. More Tips on Baby-Making Sex.   132
185. The Heat of "Pregnancy" Sex.   132
186. Explore Middle-of-the-Night Sex.   137
187. Practice Children-in-the-House Sex.   138
188. Attempt First-Thing-in-the-Morning Sex.   139
189. Great Lover Moment: The Morning Erection.   139
190. Relish Late-Afternoon Sex.   140
191. Talk Dirty to Me.   140
192. Sex in the Shower.   140
193. Sex in the Bath.   141
194. Sex in a Steam Room.   141
195. Skinny-Dip.   142
196. Have Sex Even When You're Not in the Mood.   142
197. How to Get Your Lover Hot When He or She Is Not.   142
198. Explore Erotic Books.   143
199. Read the Kama Sutra.   144
200. Explore Erotic Movies.   144
201. Feed Each Other.   145
202. Eat Cake.   146

203. Expand Your Sensuality.   146
204. Stimulate Your Sense of Smell.   147
205. Great Lover Moment: Take Your Love Away with You.   148
206. Seeing Is Believing.   148
207. Pique Your Sense of Hearing.   149
208. Great Lover Moment: Music to Make Love By.   149
209. Touch Sensation.   150
210. The Swirl.   150
211. Tantalize Your Sense of Taste.   151
212. Create a Sanctuary in the Bedroom.   151
213. Ladies, Prepare the Bed for Your Man with Cool, Crisp Sheets.   152
214. Penis Ph.D.   152
215. The Penis Effect.   153
216. Get to Know Her Essence.   153
217. Enjoy the Rest of Her Body.   154
218. Enjoy the Other Parts of His Body As Well.   154
219. The Surprise Pleasures of Anal Penetration for Him.   155
220. Help Her Catch the A-Train.   156
221. Ladies, Take Charge.   156
222. Have Sex in an Unfamiliar Place.   156
223. Have Sex When Others Are Around.   157
224. Place a Mirror in Your Bedroom.   157
225. Paint Each Other.   158
226. Ask to Be Spanked.   158
227. Give Your Lover a Scalp Massage.   159
228. Give Your Lover a Back Massage.   159
229. Know How to Wash and Brush Your Lover's Hair.   159
230. Great Lover Moment: The Magic of a Box of Sand.   160
231. Shave Him.   160
232. Shave Her Wherever She Wishes.   161
233. How to Use Lubricant and Why.   161
234. Coitus Cloths.   162
235. Keep Your Sex Life Private.   162
236. Let Sex Be Fun.   163

The Classics: Moves, Positions, and More from My Archives

237. Ode to Bryan   166
238. It Takes Three   168
239. Y-Knot   170
240. Basket Weave.   171
241. The Art of Giving Her Oral Pleasure.   173

242. Head-On or Profile?   173
243. Vary the Speed and Pressure of Your Tongue.   174
244. For the More Delicate Flowers.   174
245. The Nose Knows (AKA Face Facts).   175
246. The Kivin Method.   175
247. Big, Soft, Wet, and Warm.   177
248. Please, No Flicking.   178
249. A Tip for Sucking Her.   178
250. Tips for the Tongue-Tired.   179
251. Avoid That Crink in Your Neck.   179
252. School Days—Forming Those Letters.   180
253. The Power of Eye Contact.   180
254. The Ring and the Seal.   181
255. Don't Forget to Mind the Stepchildren.   183
256. Ladies, Strum the Frenulum.   184
257. The Ten Ways Women Can Be Stimulated to Achieve Orgasm.   185
258. #1 Clitoral   185
259. #2 Vaginal and Cervical   185
260. #3 G Spot and AFE (Anterior Fornix Erotic) Zone   186
261. #4 Urethral (U-Spot)   186
262. #5 Breast/Nipple   187
263. #6 Mouth   187
264. #7 Anal   187
265. #8 Blended/Fusion   188
266. #9 Zone   188
267. #10 Fantasy   188
268. Great Lover Moment: Cinematographers Rule.   188
269. The Fab Four of Male Orgasm.   189
270. The Eight Ways Men Orgasm.   189
271. Anal Play—Debunking the Myths.   190
272. Cleanliness Is Next to Godliness.   191
273. Relax.   191
274. Around the Globe.   191
275. #1 Female Superior   192
276. #2 Male Superior   194
277. #3 Side by Side   196
278. #4 Rear Entry—AKA Doggie Style   198
279. #5 Sitting/Kneeling   200
280. #6 Standing   203
281. Great Lover Moment: Be Your Own Judge of Arousal.   204
282. Mindful Breathing Techniques That Enhance Sexual Experience.   205
283. Exploring the Yoni and Lingam—Tantric Techniques
     of Sexual Pleasure.   205

284. The Deer Exercise for Men.   208
285. The Washcloth Trick.   210
286. Male Multiple Orgasms.   210
287. Female Multiple Orgasms.   211
288. Kegels, Kegels, and More Kegels.   212
289. The Instruments.   213
290. Great Lover Moment: Ladies, Suck Him into You.   214
291. Hip Roll, Here We Come.   214

How to Be a Great Lover in Fantasy

292. Give Yourself and Your Partner Permission to Discuss Any Fantasy.   218
293. Ask Your Partner for a Fantasy You Haven't Been Able to Voice
     in the Past.   218
294. Get in Touch with the Feeling Fueling Your Fantasy.   219
295. Give Yourself Permission to Get into Character.   220
296. Try the Domination/Submission Fantasy.   220
297. Try the Voyeuristic/Exhibitionist Fantasy.   221
298. Ménage à Trois.   221
299. Swinging.   222
300. Indulge His Dress-Up Fantasy.   222
301. The Bored Housewife and Cabana Boy.   223
302. The Prostitute and the Gentleman.   223
303. The Officer and the Gentlewoman.   224
304. Phone Sex.   225
305. "Daddy, I've Been Bad."   225
306. Innocent Schoolgirl.   226
307. Nurse Nancy and Doctor Dan.   226
308. True Lies.   227
309. From Here to Eternity.   227
310. Bull Durham.   228
311. Talk Dirty.   228
312. How to Create Your Own Fantasies.   229
313. Incorporate Toys to Expand Your Lovemaking Options.   230
314. Lubricants for You and Your Toys.   230
315. Vibrators—External/Internal.   231
316. Bondage Light.   235
317. Goodies That Vary the Senses.   235
318. Dildos.   236
319. PVC Molded Toys.   236
320. Anal Toys.   238
321. Harnesses.   239

322. Great Lover Moment: Video Cameras, Beware.   239
323. The Pearl Necklace.   240

Frequently Asked Questions and Other New Information on the Sexual Frontier

324. How Do I Know If She's Faking?   243
325. How Do I Tell My Lover That I've Been Faking?   245
326. How Can I Have an Orgasm with Intercourse?   246
327. I'm Embarrassed to Tell My Husband I Fantasize During Sex.
     Is There Anything Wrong with That?   247
328. What Is the Difference Between a Fantasy and a Fetish?   248
329. How Can I Introduce Fantasies into My Relationship?   248
330. How Can I Be Sure I Taste Okay for Oral Sex?   250
331. I Worry That My Semen Tastes Too Strong. How Can I Be Sure?   250
332. My Partner Has Trouble Remaining Erect While He Is Pleasuring
     Me. What Can I Do?   251
333. How Can I Get My Wife to Go Down on Me More Often?   251
334. How Can I Achieve a G Spot Orgasm?   252
335. I'd Really Like to Have Anal Sex More Often. How Can I Convince
     My Girlfriend/Boyfriend to Do It? Also, Why Are People So
     Interested in Anal Sex?   253
336. If She/He Wants to Use Toys, What Does That Mean?   254
337. What Is the Normal Amount of Sex per Week? My Husband
     Wants It at Least Once a Day and I'm Too Tired.   255
338. At What Age Do I Speak to My Children about Sex?   255
339. What Is Female Ejaculation?   256
340. Do All Women Ejaculate?   256
341. How Do I Suggest a New Position?   257
342. Why Does My Girlfriend Use a Vibrator?   257
343. Will Using a Vibrator Desensitize Her to My Touch?   257
344. Where Do I Find Sex Toys?   258
345. Will Toys Ever Interfere with Our Sex Life?   258
346. I Would Really Love to Have My Wife Swallow When She Gives
     Me Oral Sex; How Should I Broach the Subject?   259
347. My Husband Wants to Watch Erotic Movies Together;
     Does That Mean There Is Something Wrong with Our Sex Life?   259
348. Is It Normal for Him to Masturbate?   259
349. We Used to Have a Great Sex Life, How Do We
     Get the Spark Back?   260
350. Viagra Is Not for Everyone.   260
351. Great Lover Moment: Don't Listen to Certain Stats.   261

352. The Skinny on Pheromones. 262
353. Alabama and Sex Toys. 262
354. Infants Like Leather? 263
355. The Truth about Circumcision. 263
356. Smoking and Teenage Sex. 264
357. Seniors and Sex. 264
358. HPV Less in Circumcised Men. 265
359. Virtual Reality Sex. 265
360. Fantasies Worldwide. 265
361. Chastity Belts Are Back, Sort Of. 266
362. Intersex: More Common Than Cystic Fibrosis. 266
363. Sex As Prevention. 267
364. Birth Control Pills and Vitamin Depletion. 267
365. Birth Control: The Choices Expand. 267

Resources 271
Bibliography 283
Index 291

Acknowledgments

*Love does not consist in gazing at each other
but in looking outward together in the same direction.*
—Antoine de Saint-Exupéry

One of the first life lessons you learn in business is: No one does it alone. Whether you are strategizing your next step, running the day-to-day operations of your company, or writing a book about those operations, you can't do it without the support, guidance, and help of many. I refer to them as my teams. I couldn't have done it without them.

The Support Team
The fabulous and unique ladies in my family: Raptor, Wiz, Katerena, Natashsa (AKA Michelle Paget), and Boris (AKA Lisa Paget).

My executive assistant, Michele Thompson, and her predecessor, Tara Raucci.

To all who have been there yet again through this creative venture and I won't name names but likely some of you will see yourselves in these Tips:

Sandra Beck, Maura McAniff, Jessica Kalkin, Sherri Tenpenny, Nance Mitchell, Alan Cochran, Christian Thrasher, Kendra King, Richard Gerstein, Morley Winnick, Mike Friend and Randy Smith, Robbi Mermel, Jenny McDaniel, Tara Raucci, Bob Robinson, Mark and Scott Charbonneau, Ariel Sotolongo, Wayne Davis, Raymond Davi, Grace Evans, Eileen Michaels, Lane Hancock, Wayne and Marsha Williams, Bernard Spigner, Francisca Martinez, Craig Dellio, Gwinn Ioka, Elaine Wilkes, Paul Drill, Jacqui Brandwynne, Matthew Davidge, Rhonda Britten, Priscilla Wallace, and Frederic Goldencoat.

The Creative Team
Debra Goldstein my fabulous agent, thank you again for your vision and support.

Mary Ann Naples and Nicole Diamond Austin at the Creative Culture.

Mark Charbonneau, thank you again for *your* vision.

Lauren Marino, executive editor; Bill Shinker, publisher; and Mark Roy, assistant editor, at Gotham Books. So lovely to be working together again, you make this process easy.

Billie Fitzpatrick, my writing partner. I don't think we can get any faster.

Diego Felipe, illustrator; Lucas Mansell, copy editor; Ray Lundgren, graphic artist, for the cover; and all at Gotham Books.

Robin and Bob Park at Hollywood Webs.

The Research and Development Team
Marc Ganem, M.D.; Sherri Tenpenny, D.O.; Beverly Whipple, Ph.D.; Patti Britton, Ph.D.; Gary Richwald, M.D.; Stephen Sacks, M.D.; Jacqueline Snow, M.N., C.N.P.; John Feldsted; Rob Clink; Tom Stewart; and Violet Blue.

The Presentation Team
Lilianna and Ali Moradi, Moradi Studios, for keeping me presentable. J'ai Lone and her terric m akeup. Ron Derhacopian, for his stunning photography.

A special thank you to Dr. Marc Ganem for the artistic support, and Dr. Beverly Whipple for her proofing expertise.

Introduction

$\mathcal{A}$ little over ten years ago, I began organizing women's focus groups on the subject of sex. I wanted information about sex that was accurate, reliable, and helpful and not tied to the myths and misleading depictions of the adult-male porn industry—and I knew other women wanted this information as well. What I didn't anticipate was that my small, informal discussion groups would explode in popularity and that I would establish a new career as a sexuality educator. Suddenly dozens, then hundreds, then thousands of women and men began contacting me with the same questions I had originally raised. In order to respond to this hunger for information, I have given sexuality seminars for women, men, and couples around the world, and I have written three books, *How to Be a Great Lover*, *How to Give Her Absolute Pleasure*, and *The Big O.*

365 Days of Sensational Sex is my fourth book, and by far the most comprehensive of all of them. Like its predecessors, it came out of my work with women, men, and couples, who, like yourselves, seek and deserve the most up-to-date, accurate information there is on the subject of sexuality. This book arose out of a demand from my clients who for years have begged me to share with them the best of the best secrets from couples who are having great, ongoing sex, or who were able to reignite their passion to keep on having mind-blowing sex throughout the duration of their relationship. What is it that makes some people such great lovers, capable of having and sustaining fabulous sex and sizzling relationships? What is it these people are doing that keeps the fire burning? And most important, what secrets can I share that will enable other curious readers to become great lovers themselves?

Many people assume that being a great lover is about learning tips on technique, but that is far from the truth. Strange to hear, I am sure, from the author who has written extensively about technique, but as I've said many times before, the "what goes where" and "how to" elements of sex are only the tip of the iceberg. You can know all the parlor tricks in the world and may possibly be tons of fun when horizontal, but what makes you a great lay is not necessarily what makes you a great lover.

Defining great sex is personal and very connotative. There is no dictionary definition. For one person it might mean being able to give and receive off-the-chart orgasms, for another it might be about adventure and things you can attach to the ceiling, and for yet another it might be about feeling amazingly close and connected while wrapped in a lover's arms. But from what I have learned through my years of listening closely to people, great sex boils down to two factors:

- Great Lovers possess an attitude toward sex that is open and curious, willing to learn something new about sex—always and forever.

- Great Lovers possess the know-how and the intention to keep the flames of passion alive—always and forever.

The truth of these two factors became startlingly clear recently when Claire, a woman in her sixties, called to ask me advice on how to resuscitate her sexual relationship with her husband, Marty, also in his sixties. Recently, her husband had gone through heart-bypass surgery. On top of this medical crisis, Marty was also getting ready to retire.

Claire was feeling overwhelmed not only by her concerns for her husband's health, but for herself—how was she going to take care of him, take care of the family (she was now the main breadwinner), and take care of her job? And did I mention that her company was transferring her to the office in Las Vegas?

Claire was clearly a formidable professional and a deeply caring woman, and because of this, she was determined to finesse all these transitions in her life. One of her first tasks was to address her concerns about her sexual relationship with Marty. Before his surgery, their sex life had always been good—for thirty-five years of marriage, she pointed out to me. But now, it was virtually nonexistent. Rather than succumb to her fears that Marty was unable to have great sex anymore, Claire decided to take the bull by the horns, so to speak.

I suggested that she get my other books. I also shared with her some of the secrets contained in the following pages. To get the ball rolling, I suggested two simple-yet-powerful ways that I predicted would boost her husband's waning sexual self-confidence and get his attention (and interest) back into sex:

- First, let him know that he is still irresistible. Claire tried to make him feel how they did when they first got together by doing what she used to do in the back of his car. Claire showed Marty how much she was still attracted to him, which began to revive his sexual pulse.

- Second, use his body for your sexual pleasure. Claire tapped into how most men get turned-on: watching his lover do herself with the essence of his masculinity—his penis.

Two weeks later, at a networking group we both attended, Claire stood up proudly and acknowledged me by saying in a very strong voice, "I want you to know that you helped me put the zip and spark back into a thirty-five-year-old marriage!"

To this day, I am convinced that if Claire and Marty could, anyone can learn how to reignite the flames and give their sexual relationship a passionate longevity. Don't you want to have the kind of sex that makes you lick your lips before you have it, dream in anticipation of the event, and smile rather smugly afterward? That is what I am hoping this book will enable each and every one of you to do with these 365 tips.

Every once in a while, a client or seminar attendee will share with me a pearl of wisdom about his or her sex life or relationship that smacks so startlingly of the truth that I immediately add it to my data bank of "great lover's secrets." Over the years, I have distilled the best of the best secrets into 365 gems, which I now want to share with you. Some of the secrets are geared toward women; this information is what men want women to know about what really works for them. It is also information that women have said works for them and their men. The secrets that are directed to men are made up of information that women want men to know about what works for them, and what men have told me work for them and their lovers. In this fly-on-the-wall way, the book works like a unique conversation: women and men have equal platforms for discovering, discussing, and deciding on what to do with each other.

I want to share with you many of these truths about what people who are truly great lovers have told me: what they have done with their partners, why they have done it, how they did it, what worked or didn't work, and the ways that they were able to add spice to their sex lives; the ways they were able to keep their relationship new and fresh and as sexy and satisfying as it was on the day they met. These secrets will inspire you and your partner, in your own unique way, to give to and receive from each other mind-blowing levels of pleasure that will literally transform the sexual energy in your relationship. In short, you will learn how to keep the sizzle—forever!

The book contains 365 short entries, each one revealing a different gem of how great lovers continue to turn on their partners, maintain access to intimacy, and pave the way to take him or her to their preferred heights of pleasure. The tips are placed in the six categories that create sizzling sex for Great Lovers: Attitude, Behavior, Playbook (new tips and techniques), Classics (favorite tips and techniques from my seminars), Fantasy, and Frequently Asked Questions. Within these categories you will find suggestions on how you can apply these tried-and-true methods to your own relationships. You will also come across Great Lover Moments, provocative real-life stories that will not only whet your mental whistle, but will also shed light on the inner workings of the best relationships with which I have had the privilege of working.

These tips pertain directly to how sex invigorates your entire relationship. I have seen firsthand that truly dynamite sex comes not just from technique, but from mastering the secrets that get to the underlying dynamics of relationships. Some of these secrets may at first seem like common sense, but one thing I've learned is that when it comes to keeping the charge of intimacy, common sense isn't all that commonly practiced. You might think you know all the basics—like learning how to move the target on her pleasure, the ten ways in which a woman can orgasm, or using all of your senses to seduce your man—but are you putting this information into play? What I hope to do here is make these secret tips work for you, by giving you what I call the W-5: the Who, What, Where, When, and Why these tips worked for my clients and in doing so have them work for you. Who knows? You may suddenly look at some of these pieces of "common sense" in a whole new way.

This is not a book about how to fix a relationship that is broken, nor is it about comparing yourself to others to see if you measure up. There are plenty of books out there that want to do that. This book is all about making something good, great; something great, sensational. In essence, this book makes five promises:

- You will find fresh and sexy concrete tips that will enable you to drive your lover wild with desire and deliver even greater satisfaction to you because you can do so.

- You will validate your own sexual experiences, be able to expand on them as you hear about how others navigate their relationships, deepen their bonds, and increase the sexual energy between them.

- You will discover your full sexual potential by exploring new forms of pleasure and new ways to connect with your partner, again and again.

- You will know how other long-term couples regularly access the pulse-quickening sex of their early encounters, and how that too can be yours.

- And you will absolutely learn what keeps the passion passionate!

You don't necessarily have to be in a relationship right now to benefit from this book. You may want to simply use the book as a resource and guide for when the right lady or gentleman finally does come along in your life. As humans, we are all phenomenally social creatures; indeed, it is in our nature to want to be in relationships. So even if you're not in a relationship now, you are probably thinking about the one you'd like to be in. Whether you are single or have been with the same person for twenty years, let these 365 tips be your guide, your wish list, and your inspiration. This little book is my gift to you—the essential gems that will give you the key to keeping your relationship humming, as if the honeymoon had never ended.

How to Be a Great Lover in Attitude

It's best we start at the very beginning. Plainly said, Great Sex begins with a specific attitude toward sex, an attitude that is open toward sex, comfortable with sex, and desirous of sex. Put simply, a Great Lover always wants to know more about sex, and this attitude is like an internal compass that guides them, inspires them, and soothes them. They understand the power of their sexuality and know how to extend this to their lover. This power is what shapes their attitudes—toward sex, their lovers, and themselves. In this section, you will learn how to hone your Great Lover attitude, shape it, or refresh your memory (or that of your lover) of why it's so important to having Great Sex.

1. Falling-in-Love Sex vs. Being-in-Love Sex.

Allow that falling-in-love sex is different from being-in-love sex. Anyone who has ever fallen in love knows it is a dizzying experience that takes over your life and brain. According to Dr. Helen Fisher, there is a true physiological response associated with falling in love, and yet so many people complain that inevitably the white-hot heat slacks off. Well in a way, thank goodness—or we'd stay in that state forever and get little done. Joking aside (and I'm not really joking), most people reminisce about the great sex they used to have, despairing that it disappears when the honeymoon ends. Does the passion have to end? No. And you now have 365 ways to prove that to be true.

Real, authentic falling-in-love sex not only continues to exist, but can be tapped into for years to come. In order for you to benefit from this awareness, you need to accept that as your relationship grows and matures, your bond will deepen, naturally changing the headiness of falling-in-love sex into the deeper passion of being-in-love sex.

At some point in your relationship, you have to accept that the future brings changes and these changes will impact your sexual relationship. Great Lovers know that the secret for transforming falling-in-love sex into being-in-love sex is learning how to go with the flow by adapting your expectations and broadening the range of what is possible to please each other. With that greater variety to choose from, you will have more options to access sexual pleasure in whatever way that works for you. As Sheila says, "Yes, our sex is different. But it's also deeper and more spiritual and more erotic. Not the quarry but the chase, not the trophy but the race."

2. Sex Beyond Intercourse.

You need to accept that great, loving sex isn't only about intercourse. What I have heard consistently in ten years is that intercourse is but one segment of great lovemaking—especially for those couples who are not physically able to have intercourse due to pain, illness, or injury. Now, I am in no way taking away from intercourse as a terrific part of sex, but I am pointing out that if you rely only on intercourse as the way of being sexual with your lover, then you seriously limit your mutual ability for sexual pleasure. As the tips and techniques of this book show, there is a smorgasbord of pleasurable activities out there to turn on you and your partner, and you can pick and choose from them and combine them in countless ways. Remember what Dr. Bernie Zilbergeld, the author of *The New Male Sexuality,* said, "One specific action alone does not define our lovemaking; intercourse is only a part of our sexual experience."

3. Give Yourselves Permission.

Permission is a huge component of healthy sexuality, both the giving and the receiving of it. And often, the biggest gift givers of permission are our very selves. Given that sexuality is the place where we all begin, it's amazing that we humans culturally give ourselves so little permission to know and to not know about our sexuality. This is our most powerful form of communicating; it is what creates life and love and every one of us. I am not going to go into why as a culture we grant each other so little permission to know, learn, and experience sexuality, but what I will address is that there are ways to circumvent this no-permission acculturation in your relationship. Great Lovers know that permission authorizes and gives them and their partners space in which to discuss and explore everything from their own experiences (how to orgasm in more than one way) to what they'd like to try (playing out fantasies) to what they've always been curious about (toys). For Great Lovers, the permission that exists in their intimate relationship has an "I won't judge what you say" attitude, and has been the ticket for them as a couple to go to another level of sexual heat.

Men and women often arrive at relationships thinking that they should already know everything there is about sex. Nothing could be further from the truth. So before going any further—in your relationship or in the reading of this book—stop and give yourselves permission to not know. What happens next? You open yourselves to learning some of the most sensational, sizzling tips about sex you will ever encounter.

4. Know There Is Always More to Know about Sex.

This will be one of the few times I use myself as an example. People will often say "You must know everything about sex." And my response very honestly is "No, I don't. I learn and hear something new about sexuality every day, and the reason I do is because I have the attitude that there is *always* more to learn about everything in life, sex included." I may hear about a new study being considered, read a definition I didn't know, hear a new way of asking a question, attend a trade show and see new products, hear field researchers explain new ways of using products, discover a new component for novelties, learn about a better source for products, a variation on a position, a suggestion of how to clarify X, Y, or Z descriptions, or comments from peers on how to hone discussion points. The beauty of having an openness to any subject is that you can approach it with a "new" attitude, every time. And what better area to have an open attitude than sexuality? Even if you've been in the same relationship for many years, you can learn something new and surprise your partner or go somewhere sexually that you've never gone before. You just need to open yourself up to the possibility and allow yourself to be curious.

5. Treat Her Like a Lady.

Gentlemen, this tip may sound like a throwback to another era. Let me make this perfectly clear: there is nothing more powerful, nothing more of a turn-on than if you treat your lover as a lady. What does this mean? Be a gentleman. This entails doing things gentlemen should do: opening car doors, holding doors open, letting her on and off the elevator first, helping a woman on with her coat, and rising when she gets back to the table. Women need to be acknowledged by your good manners. It will make them feel more feminine and see you as more masculine. Honest. Gentlemen, women know that your behaving well and having manners are part of the dance of seduction, and your actions will invariably result in increasing your odds of becoming intimate or having sex.

6. Gentlemen, Let Her Know You Want to Make Her Come— Anytime, Anywhere, Anyhow.

This tip is not about learning technique, nor is it about your performance. This tip is all about how much pleasure a woman experiences when she knows her lover loves to make her come. Quite simply, gentlemen, it's up to you to let your woman know you are enjoying yourself as you are pleasuring her. This will let her relax, feel taken care of and loved. If she thinks you are uncomfortable, she will feel uncomfortable. Whether you tell her flat out, "Baby, I'll take you there!" or whether she knows by virtue of your sheer determination and will, you need to let your desire for her shine forth clearly. Men have told me that there is no more powerful an aphrodisiac than being able to bring a woman to orgasm; and that alone is a beautiful thing. But it's important to remember, gentlemen, not to get caught up in your performance. Rather, focus on freeing yourself to roam her body as you chart the endless territory of her sensuality. As you will read later in this book, women can experience orgasms in ten different ways. It's up to you to discover or enhance your approach shots. There is no right or wrong way, there is only the intention to elicit her pleasure. And by all means, try to enjoy yourself.

One woman, Terry, had been married for almost six years before her husband, Michael, gave her oral sex. Why did he wait? Because he was afraid that she didn't want him to go down on her. Finally, after Terry attended one of my women's seminars, she realized that she should just bring up the subject, so she asked Michael if he had an "aversion" to giving her oral sex. He was flabbergasted. "An aversion," he cried, "I've been wanting to do that all these years. I thought you didn't like it! You never asked for it!" Talk about time-is-a-wasting! The point: Don't assume, simply ask.

7. Ladies, Remember That Oral Sex Isn't Just for Dating.

First, let me say that throughout your relationship your desire to do many sexual acts will change, rather like the phases of the moon, waxing and waning with time. And, as with anything intimate, what works for one couple won't necessarily work for another. Having said that, I feel compelled to include this Be-careful-you-don't-fall-into comment. In over a decade of talking to people, many couples have shared with me how certain parts of sex were great *before* marriage or commitment, but that *after* marriage or commitment, or moving in together, this specific act or even sex simply stops. This is often the case with oral sex, especially women giving it to men. Some of this slacking off of women giving oral sex to men is similar to why couples stop kissing: The comfort zone of relationships is a breeding ground for complacency. Secondly, *some* women tend to think of giving oral sex as a "have to" instead of a "want to." Let me share with you a cautionary tale, one that captures the cynical extreme of this situation.

In one noteworthy seminar I heard the two following comments: "My husband only gets a BJ once a year on his birthday. Yeah, I did it more when we were dating, but not anymore." The follow-up comment from another attendee on her friend's change of "desire" was, "Hey, you already have the kids and the house in Bel-Air, you don't have to do it anymore anyway." Now, these two women may not be typical in their cynicism, but they do present a very concrete example of women who stop sharing oral sex with their men.

Ladies, after ten years of listening to men, I must share with you that men say that ceasing to give or offer oral sex that was once part of your regular sexual repertoire is "Just not okay." This rule of the bedroom goes back to a very basic way men think about their masculinity: they want to feel sexually desired and taken care of by their partners, and for the majority of men, oral sex is one of the surest ways to accomplish this. Your job, then, is to get in touch with your desire to give your lover pleasure, which will then get you in touch with *your* pleasure. For Great Lovers, the two go hand in hand. And for the record, men don't seem to encounter the same problem: They continue to give oral sex to women long into their relationships. Why? They enjoy it!

8. Let Him Be the Man.

Ladies, the more feminine you are, the more masculine he can be. And the more you honor and sustain his masculinity, the more primal the sexual energy between you. Great Lovers know there is nothing androgynous or asexual about their being sexual, and they revel in and enjoy their given sexuality. The more you are in your power sexually as a woman, the more space and permission there is for him to be in his power sexually as a man. This truth is connected to the oft-unspoken concept that women control the access to sex and its activities: Hence, the more you allow yourself to be the woman in the relationship, the more you allow him to be the man. This subtle but powerful dynamic was captured by one international female entrepreneur in this way: "In day-to-day business I do it all, yet when I am with my fiancé, I can be as soft and as feminine as I feel, which is as much a reflection of his masculinity as it is of my own femininity. I know my femininity by how masculine he is, in public and in private." So what does this look like? This isn't about a male tough-guy thing, it's about socio-cultural mirroring from bygone eras. Women who are Great Lovers have an innate expression and mastery of their femininity that makes their men feel as if they are the proverbial "King of the World." I know this may sound hackneyed and clichéd, but this concept walks hand and hand with the adage, "Lady in the parlor; harlot in the boudoir." This is about social differences between women and men, the doors, the manners, and the social niceties. The more a man and a woman have the awareness of those social niceties outside the bedroom, the more there can be a sexual difference in the bedroom. Many men have shared with me that there are few things that get their motors running more than feminine women: "It is how I know I am a man. Look, when I am out with my wife I want to be with a woman all the other men want. Shallow? Nope.

I am telling you how men really think." This tip speaks to the splendid dichotomy and difference between the sexes. The more feminine the woman on a man's arm, the more masculine he appears, and goodness knows men strive to appear masculine and powerful.

9. Stay Current.

This tip involves defining your sexual experience by whom you are with now, not on past experiences or relationships. Few of us are virgins when we arrive at our ultimate relationship. Yet, no man or woman likes to be reminded of that fact or have our histories reexamined. We tend to appreciate the skills learned in former ties, but we don't like to be made aware of how those skills may have been learned. That said, it's up to you to make your current relationship the one that is most sexually satisfying. It's easy, when referencing other relationships—good or bad—to stray mentally, emotionally, or physically from the one you're in. Even the slightest thought can take you away from the now. So give your memory of past events their due by allowing them to teach and guide you, and don't get stuck comparing and contrasting the old with the new.

10. Vulnerability = Value.

Our vulnerabilities show us and the world where others can make a contribution to us, where by virtue of another being there for us they make a difference in our lives. The take-away of this statement is "People stay in your life mentally or physically when they feel they are making a contribution to you." When there isn't a place or space for them to show up for you, they don't. Your vulnerabilities are often the first and most sensitive area in which they can do so. You know yourself that when you can be there for someone, especially someone near and dear to your heart, there is a very real physical feeling of satisfaction when you've done something good. And it is increased even more so because of their importance to you.

Just a little tip here, invariably the last thing you want people to know about you is one of the first things they become aware of, whether you say it or not. If you are really very shy, but think acting aloof will make you appear more secure, think again. People will know. And the truest parts of you are the most appealing to people *because* they are that real. Does it feel comfy at first to let people know what you think, to see you warts and all? Will that make you unacceptable or not okay? No, but then growth and change in relating isn't always comfy either, and the more open you are to sharing your softer sides, the more the important person in your life is likely to protect that sensitive flank. Why? Because when you are someone's someone, that sensitive flank is theirs, too. Just remember, Great Lovers are unafraid of being vulnerable.

11. The Legacy of Trusting.

Trusting your lover is a gift that you and *only* you can give to him or her. Trust creates an ongoing legacy within your relationship. So what does this legacy look like? In your bedroom, trust is the foundation that allows other parts of your love life to flourish and develop. This is the single most commonly cited trait that Great Lovers say makes their relationships and sexual heat continue. Simply said, they trust each other in and out of the bedroom. They trust themselves and they trust their relationships. This incredibly valuable and fragile gift is earned and treated gently and ongoingly by those couples with satisfying and thriving relationships. And these couples often say trusting is neck and neck with respecting their partner and relationship.

12. Relationship As Refuge.

Just as your bedroom is your sanctuary, your relationship is your refuge—from work commitments, family obligations, and life's responsibilities in general. Your relationship should be the anchor in the middle of your life, giving you support and a tether, while at the same time enough rope to grow, learn, and live. Couples who have established this feeling say it enables them to do so much more in their lives—in all areas of their lives. It goes without saying that the more relaxed and less frenetic you are in any situation, the more you can get done and the better you are at what you do. When your relationship is a haven, I have heard again and again partners describe this haven as full of support, a safety net, and as "contentedness." As one man from a couple's seminar said, "I like to come home and feel like the world is on the outside. Once I'm home, I always know she is on my team." Given all the stresses we place on ourselves, and let's be honest, we create much of this stress ourselves, couples who create this ambience when they are together enhance and inspire each other mentally and physically, inside and outside the boundaries of their relationship. And no matter how cold it may be outside, you always know that the emotional place you and your lover created inside when you came together is there, waiting for you to return to—for succor, a sense of peace, and, of course, sex.

13. Intellectual Freedom.

Some couples are immediately drawn to each other intellectually. At their first meeting, they fall into swift and deep discussions of favorite films, books, or philosophers. They move from discussions to outings and ultimately to the bedroom. Others of us aren't as apparently lucky, and it takes longer to establish such vital brain energy in the relationship. Which doesn't mean it's difficult—creating an intellectual connection can be as easy as choosing a movie to see, enjoying it together, and then talking about it afterward. And when you create an intellectual camaraderie with your partner, you are adding another dimension to your relationship. The camaraderie comes from exchanging ideas with each other; this mental stimulation not only keeps your brains awake, it also keeps them engaged with each other's brains. Haven't you ever wondered what he really thinks? Don't you wish she would have an opinion that surprised you? This kind of back and forth not only adds excitement to your relationship, it also keeps you on your toes: No one will say you've become as boring as an old pair of slippers. And how does this intellectual energy stimulate your sex life? Exactly as you might imagine: your intellect kick-starts your most powerful sexual organ, your brain, making your lover more interesting and exciting. Ergo, you have heightened the lust factor!

14. Cherish.

If you want to avoid the pitfall of focusing on the negative instead of the positive in your relationship, then you need to cherish the qualities you love in your partner. At first, this tip may seem kind of blasé, but hear me out: When we get used to our lover's presence in our lives, and begin to get comfortable, there's often a shift into the negative. We tend to focus more on the qualities of our lover that we don't necessarily like. Why? Because we get disconnected from that falling-in-love energy, where all we did was focus on the good in our partner. So here's my advice: Pay conscious attention to those qualities in your partner that you like, love, appreciate, respect, and admire. That, my dears, is the definition of "cherish."

15. Love vs. Lust.

When we first meet and fall in love, there is very little distinction between loving and lusting. We flow from lust to love effortlessly—all sexual encounters seemed infused with love and all moments of love (exchanges of loving energy) are touched by lust. But as our relationships mature, growing more solid roots, we tend to separate love and lust, making them distinct and hard to commingle. We do this unconsciously, but we do it all the same. And when this separation occurs, you needlessly add stress around love and lust. As Great Lovers, you need to know two things: 1) that like good wine, relationships must age to bear the fruit of abundant flavor. Such aging means resisting this tendency to separate love and lust; and 2) that all you need to know how to do is keep the flow between these two components open. Some nights, sex may be all about lust, with the two of you tearing off each other's clothes and making love on the kitchen island. Some mornings, you might look at each other across the pillows and smile, knowing the *deep* love between you. You come together without words, but in total love. Great Lovers know that it's the synergy between love and lust that sustains a relationship—sexually and emotionally. So try to become comfortable with the interplay between love and lust, and you will learn how to move seamlessly from the heat of lust into the passion of lovemaking—sometimes within the same embrace. Nowhere is it written that you must have the same ambience and attitude throughout an evening of lovemaking—that would be like asking you to maintain the same dance step all night.

16. Stand Up for Your Rights.

Take responsibility for your rights within the relationship. Now, this tip is not about flat-out entitlement; it's about a permission granted and understood by virtue of your commitment to each other. As such, these rights, like little plants, require tending and nurturing. What rights am I referring to? The right to ask where you were and where you are going. There is also the right of one partner to request the other partner to wear something more "suitable" in public. It's also the right of a partner to inquire about the other's work situation and offer his or her opinion. I am not suggesting that it is all right for one person to try to control the other person. Rather, I am stating that it is perfectly understandable and expected for you both to get involved in any aspect of each other's lives that impacts the relationship. These rights are often unspoken statements about how you show you care about the "us" of your relationship.

Everyone wants to know they are safe even when not together. These rights, like respect and trust, are acquired and earned. One of the best examples I have to illustrate the power of this tip was a girlfriend who in the first month of dating a man received a call from him at 11 P.M. Her indignant response to me while we were on the phone at 11:30 P.M. was "It is entirely too early for him to be calling that late." I collapsed laughing and asked, "So when would it not be too early?" She was very clear about when the right to call late would be granted in a relationship with her. So as funny as such "rules" may be, they have a serious side, and it's about respecting personal boundaries. And Great Lovers pay close attention to such arbitrarily granted privileges.

17. Sowing Roots.

Be close and stay close in order to sow deep roots for the intimacy that leads to Great Sex. I'm talking about emotional territory here, and some of us are more fluent and comfortable with our emotions than others. But it's necessary for all of us to work at being close and staying close. This means continuing to ask how each other's day was, how you feel about X, Y, or Z. It's up to you to make sure you know how your partner feels about life in general, your relationship, and your life together. Inquire. Listen. Offer feedback. Care about how he or she is doing. Don't wait until an issue arises, a crisis breaks out, or an unbearable silence begins to prevail over the household. The ability and potential to always have Great Sex relies on many things, but one crucial factor is a couple's ability to be close and stay close.

18. Frequency Is Dynamic.

Like the daily ebb and flow of tides, there is a natural cycle of sexual frequency in most relationships. I know of some lovers who relish the change in how often they have sex because when they vary their frequency, they also vary the where and the how of sex. Such lovers are displaying a glass-half-full attitude about frequency variation. They are confident in their need to take a break, knowing that when they resume relating, they can either re-create what they were doing before or try something new and different.

19. A Calm Before the Storm.

Invariably we see relationships on television and in films depicted as being tumultuous and dramatic, with people dashing hither, thither, and yon. Great Lovers know a different truth about a relationship that combines reality with a slow, sexual simmer. Consider this: Can you describe how you knew you were in love? Many times I have asked long-term couples how they knew this was the "real thing." And almost without fail, they have stated that they experienced an immediate, calm knowingness that infused them, and the entire relationship. As one woman said, "There was no noise in my brain and there was a calm in my heart." This calmness speaks to the belief and truth in that feeling with an intangible certainty that defies description. When Great Lovers first meet, they invariably say there was "a stillness" in which "nothing but they existed." Thank goodness we listen to that tiny voice because we then get to reap the rewards of stillness: the sexual storm that follows.

20. Relish How Your Body Makes Your Lover Feel.

"To me from me" is how a Canadian woman describes the emotional synergy she creates for herself, knowing her body and actions make her lover so bananas. Truly, you are the only one who can bask in the post-coital glow of your lover. And only you can know the satisfaction of making your lover feel that good. So the next time you make love, linger in the afterglow and relish how your body made your lover wild with pleasure.

21. Are You Willing to Talk Dirty?

Did your eyebrows just arch? Anytime you let yourself try new things and experiment, you are exercising an open attitude toward sex. This tip is meant to encourage you to be willing to experiment with explicit language in public. Now, there is no need to do (or say) anything you're not comfortable with. Yet consider how you feel when you put on a new outfit? In the same way that something on the outside can evoke those "I'm hot" feelings, so too can something from the inside. Consider starting with some of these lab exercises:

- Privately deliver (i.e. whisper) explicit language in public where you can't act on your comment

- For the ladies in the audience, as you are completing your final touch of lipstick, consider rouging your nipples, or around your other lips if you like to trim that tender area, and then tell him you've done so once you are out the door.

22. Are You Open to Enhancers?

Couples who are open to enhancers invariably discover a whole new, fun side to their sexual relationship, filled with heightened sensations and new intensities. Many times people think enhancers are simply toys. They also assume that toys only come in one form and do only one thing: phalluses that vibrate. Indeed many are and do but even more of them aren't and don't. That bottle of almond oil nestled next to the balsamic vinegar can enhance the flow of hands over a body with as much ease as it can create taste sensations for your next salad. The real beauty of these products is that they enhance sensation and we have five senses we can target. Make a list of all five senses and then create the things you'd like to try. Is it aromatherapy? Do you want to see if using jasmine essential oil in your bath does prove aphrodisiacal for you? Perhaps patchouli is your partner's favorite. Will oysters enhance your sex drive or is chocolate more your preference? Which visual treat does it for you? Which style of visual—book, video, or live lap dance? In the auditory category, what music do you like to listen to when you dine at the dining room table? Would you play the same CD while you are *on* the dining room table? Using your five senses as your guide (and there is more information on that topic in the Playbook, Tips 203–211), begin to explore how you might use enhancers to increase your pleasure. In the Fantasy section, you will find a complete up-to-date listing of many toys from which to choose.

23. Great Lover Moment: Great Lovers Are Shrewd Consumers.

As I give you a tip on being open to sexual enhancers of all types, I also would be remiss if I did not caution you against the many untested, potentially harmful products out there. The importance of this tip was driven home recently when I received a call from a marketing representative asking me to add a new product to my line. When I asked her if any research had been done, she simply said, "It takes too long to research women." You can imagine my response. Here are some fairly recent products you should be aware of:

- ViaCream—a mentholated petroleum product that is applied topically and supposedly increases a woman's libido and sexual responsiveness. This was created using Viagra's research. The manufacturers infer that what works for men when they use Viagra also works for women, with no published research to support their product's claim.

- Enzyte—a product that supposedly increases penis size and makes him last longer.

- Her Turn—another product that promises to increase a woman's libido and enhance sexual responsiveness, but its Web site offers no further research data on the product itself.

- Avlimil—a sage supplement that supposedly "corrects" female sexual dysfunction, again no published research.

In general, you should always read labels very carefully and if you have any questions, call the company. Consider these steps:

- check to see if they have published their research results in reputable peer-review journals—if they have done proper double-blind placebo-controlled studies in which their results can be replicated

- do your homework and see if the marketers have taken a grain of truth from other studies and built a beach

- check to see who the test-audience was

Be aware that slick marketing companies want you to use their products so that you can make your sex life better. But Great Lovers know that if they do try a certain product, they don't try it again if they encounter no results, any irritation, or harm. Remember, it's your body, so be sure you know what is being used on it and in it.

24. Be Brave Enough to Share Your Innermost Fantasies.

As you will see later on, I offer an abundance of tips on how to add a component of fantasy, or explore one, into your sex life. But before you look at those rather explicit tips, you must be ready in spirit: Are you brave enough to share your innermost fantasy? The one that gets you hot when you lie in bed alone, but that you've been too shy about voicing to your lover? Those of you who have summoned the courage know the incredible freedom and exhilaration that comes from the sharing alone—never mind what comes from the sharing. No fantasy is that outrageous. No fantasy is that original. But the fear comes from not knowing how your partner may react or from imagining that she or he will be turned off. However, if you have two things in place, then you can access your courage quite directly: 1) You must have faith and trust in your partner. I'm assuming this trust is already in place; 2) You must have faith and trust in yourself that you can ask for this.

25. Be Willing to Change Something about Your Appearance to Suit Your Lover's Preference.

This secret is premised on the shared goal of creating and adding to the sexual energy between the two of you. If he likes you to wear your hair down because it gets him totally excited, then it's not too much to do for that added excitement. One woman told me that her husband gets totally horny when she paints her fingernails dragon red. "He visualizes them wrapped around 'Little Tim.'" Need I say more? As always, I'm not suggesting that you do anything that makes you uncomfortable, but rather a small adjustment that may make all the difference to him or her. One woman just loves to play with the curling hair at the nape of her lover's neck. So when he goes to the barber, he simply requests that the barber not take off "too much off the back. She likes to play with it." By the barber's trimming less, he gets more. So why does this work for Great Lovers? Because in agreeing to modify something for your partner, you are making an unspoken yet loud declaration that you have heard your lover's opinion and it is important to you. You are showing your lover that you are willing to do something to please him or her. Perhaps this is why, over a period of time, Great Lovers begin to resemble one another in appearance; however, I personally draw the line at matching bowling shirts and sweaters.

26. Be Willing to Listen to Your Lover's Complaints about You.

Again, none of us is perfect. So it makes sense that we can annoy, disappoint, or hurt our partners on occasion. Hopefully, we are not doing any of this misbehaving on purpose, but rather because we are perhaps unconscious or distracted by other things in our hectic lives. But when it comes time for your partner to air his or her grievances, it's crucial that you listen without talking back, without defending yourself, and without justifying your actions or behavior. A tidy, humble, and heartfelt explanation of why can only come after you have fully listened to your mate, acknowledged his or her hurt feelings, and thought about how the event occurred. The importance of your partner voicing things is *your listening*. Remember, you cannot lead unless you listen, and when your partner feels heard, this listening often leads straight to the bedroom.

27. Be Gentle When Airing a Disappointment or Hurt Caused by Your Partner.

When it is your turn to air such a grievance, try to be thoughtful, making sure you are speaking from the point of view of how the action or behavior has made you feel, not from the perspective of trying to make your partner feel guilty. The point you are trying to make is to show your lover how they hurt or disappointed you and give them the opportunity to apologize and change or stop the egregious behavior. If you deliver your message in an angry or hateful tone, then all your lover is going to hear is the anger and hate; they will never hear your hurt, your desire for an apology, and your love. And FYI, ladies, men do not want to be around angry women, in the same way women do not want to be around angry men. Not that you can't have your moments, but you do need to know that a steady diet of anger may cause you to lose a lot of weight—mainly him.

28. Practice Approaching Your Partner from a Point of View of Mutual Respect, Not Blame or Defensiveness.

Great Lovers strive to approach one another from the platform of mutual respect, which requires a kind and gentle approach even in times of anger, frustration, or disappointment. This platform of mutual respect is one of the core values of Great Lover relationships. Why? Mutual respect is synergistic and innately connects you, whereas blame and defensiveness keep two people separate. When you as a couple let yourselves focus on who is at fault, you feed into a cycle of blame and defensiveness, which can take on its own downward energy spiral. On the other hand, when you show mutual respect for each other, you create an upward energy cycle that leads to resolution.

29. *The Gift of Giving.*

Sexually, for many couples the adage "It is better to give than to receive" is not a simple truism, rather it is an attitude and sexual behavior that allows them to feel their prowess as lovers and to connect more powerfully. For clarity's sake, let me explain it this way: Unless you are able to give as a lover, you are not likely to be able to access the intense physical connection of Great Lovers. A major type-A stockbroker described it as follows: "There is nothing, flat-out nothing that makes me feel more like a man than knowing I can create and give her that much pleasure. No amount of money, no business deal can make me feel like that."

30. *The Richness of Receiving.*

Despite the attitude that women are able to receive jewelry and other goodies with ease, they often have trouble receiving sexually. Why? There is still a cultural attitude that a woman is "selfish" or "demanding" if she expects her lover to pleasure her sexually. However, nothing could be further from the truth, especially according to men. The number one thing a man wants is for a woman to be open to him and sex, to receive him. When I say this in seminars, sometimes people look at me like I'm crazy. Receive? How? Receive what? To get the gist of this tip, think of an old-fashioned sense of sex and receiving, and it will make more sense. In bygone times, one spoke of being open to receive your lover in your arms, to receive their words, their caress, to receive them in your bed, into your body. Somehow, many women have lost this simple but powerful art of receiving. Clearly, from a functional standpoint a woman can and does receive her man: She receives him into her body. However, Great Lovers know that receiving is not simply a physical action; it's also psychological, emotional, and spiritual. So, ladies, when you are making love to your man, receive him as if your body were a vessel for him to luxuriate in. Extend yourself to him in love and in passion, and let him know what pleasure he brings you by being able to receive him in this way. And when you are outside of the bedroom, receive the gifts he offers, his kiss on your cheek, or his arm around your waist in the same spirit of openness and appreciation. For Great Lovers know that the secret synergy of giving and receiving is that you can't have one without the other.

31. Great Sex Is Chronologically Ageless.

As a lover you need to accept that love and sex have nothing to do with age. I love Dr. Bernie Zilbergeld's comment that all the actions of a twenty- to twenty-five-year-old are the same sexual activities of an eighty-five-year-old. Great Sex is a possibility at any age, and actually age gives one an advantage because of more experience. Despite the depiction of Great Sex occurring only between flawless young bodies, any lover with a scintilla of awareness of his or her own prowess knows that though there may have been something amazing and grand about first-time sex and hard, young bodies, young and hard do not translate into great unless there are other factors. Well maybe great for a period of time, but that alone won't sustain longevity. So whether it is a confidence or sensitivity or your ability to tie a cherry stem in a knot with your tongue, your date of birth is immaterial to your ability to create and enjoy fabulous sex. Accept that love and sex have nothing to do with age. As Dr. Bernie Zilbergeld said, Great Lovers know that great loving sex can happen just as easily at eighteen as at eighty-five. Perhaps an older body is not as vigorous or quite as responsive, but our bodies can remain sexually active as long as we remain relatively physically healthy and willing.

32. Great Lover Moment: "I Still Completely Dig Her."

My girlfriend's father still walks in the door at the end of his workday and calls to his wife of forty years, "Jane, would you mind coming here please?" And off they go to their bedroom—sometimes even in the middle of the day. I asked my girlfriend (she's one of six children) what the magic was for her parents. Her comment was, "My dad still completely digs my mom." My friend then went on to relate that as kids they knew that when the bedroom door was closed, under no circumstances were they to bother their parents. I take this GLM as proof positive that when there is a will, there is a way to fit sex into even the busiest of lives or households. So if you want to keep the sexual pilot light on, make sex a priority—no matter how many kids you have and how many years you've been together.

33. The Crying Connection.

Tears and sex have two main traits in common: They both are hot, wet, and the result of emotion. As some lovers well know, incredibly intense sex can result in intense tears. Tears show our most sensitive, soft hidden parts, the places where we are touched and impacted the most intensely. When you genuinely cry in front of or with your partner, you are giving your lover an unspoken message of how special he or she is to you. So whether the tears are caused by the stresses of work, an emotional blow, or the cat-food tin landing upside down on your new shoe, shed your tears. They are as much an outlet of emotion as an inroad in for your partner. As Dinah Shore said, "Trouble is a part of your life, and if you don't share it, you don't give the person who loves you enough chance to love you enough."

34. Touch Your Lover's Heart and Soul.

We love each other for reasons that we are often unaware of and often have difficulty articulating. But when we learn how to touch our lover's heart and soul, we not only expose our deeply seductive side, we also deepen our connection. This is especially true and powerful when we do something out of the blue, surprising our lover. A spontaneous action can literally create a power line from your heart to hers or vice versa. There are times when a lover does something that is the tiniest, simplest of things, and yet that little thing touches a partner's heart and soul. Other times, the heart-winning gesture is something so planned and so thought-out that a partner cannot believe that his or her lover has done that something *for* them. This is the operative sentence here: Great Lovers who have exceptional awareness of what touches all parts of their partner know how to bring their partners the greatest degree of joy and pleasure.

Knowing how to touch your lover physically is certainly an important zone. But I'm speaking here about learning how to touch the emotional pulse of your partner, their heart and soul. Here's one example: Greg was a band manager whose lead vocalist, Sandy, became the love of his life one certain holiday when she turned into the Good Grinch who transformed his feelings about Christmas. Sandy loved Christmas, but Greg was a borderline Scrooge. Okay, maybe he was Scrooge: He hated the holidays with a passion because his father had died during this period in the past. Greg's mood slump made it difficult for Sandy to revel in the holidays, as she always had done while growing up. But being a creative type and not one to shrink at a challenge, Sandy decided to try to change Greg's mind. She laid down some rules: They could only spend $20.00 each (in keeping with Greg's Scrooge-like tendencies), and they had to declare what they wanted. Greg told Sandy he wanted something in leather. On Christmas morning, Sandy presented

Greg with a Charlie Brown Christmas tree, complete with no ornaments and bare branches, and a cassette recorder and a letter. The letter
contained instructions that told him to play the tape and follow the directions to find twelve hidden decorations. On the tape, Sandy sang
Greg her favorite Christmas carols, beginning with "The Twelve Days
of Christmas." Each ornament that Greg then discovered in the treasure hunt contained an adjective that described a quality she loved
about him; it also contained a clue that led him to his next ornament.
When all twelve ornaments were decorating the little tree, Greg was
then instructed to open his present from Santa: a fantasy garment made
of pleather for Sandy to wear for Greg's pleasure. As hot as their evening
became, and as hot as their sex life continued to be, Greg told me that
what made that one night so unbelievable was the awareness of him
that Sandy's gift demonstrated. "She knew how to touch me at my
core," he said. "I now share why she loves Christmas."

35. Insisting on Being Right Can Kill Your Sex Life and Threaten Your Relationship.

A relationship always contains two voices and no one voice is more important than the other. This mutuality is vital to the healthy give and
take of any relationship that comes when two people are really communicating with each other. When this spirit of mutuality is disrupted—
when someone *has* to be right—you become polarized and that in turn
creates an abyss between the couple, shifting the balance and the couple's receptivity to each other. When one or both of you insists on being right, you immediately begin to drive the other person away. Ruth
and John, married for eight years, always had a healthy relationship.
Both of them have strong personalities (they're both lawyers) and were
comfortable sharing their opinions. Like Mary Matalin and James
Carville, they weren't afraid of verbal jousting—in fact, they admit that
the slightly combative energy seemed to spark great sex. Until John
struck it rich, literally. John made a killing on a tech stock, won a mas-

sive lawsuit, and was promoted to partner in his law firm all at once. Overnight, the money started rolling in and so did his "I'm always right" attitude. According to Ruth, John seemed to get carried away with his change in monetary status and he started associating his increase in earnings with his personal power. Very soon after, the dynamic of their relationship changed. "No matter what the topic of conversation," explains Ruth, "he had to be right. He was on a power trip. But hardest of all was that he stopped listening to me. And I stopped having sex with him. It was the only thing I could do." By insisting on only his viewpoint and refusing to hear his wife's voice, John undermined their mutuality and upset the delicate balance of power in the relationship. This simple act had the power to push Ruth away in one instant. Sadly, those two are still in a relationship stalemate. In order to avoid this common pitfall of intimate relationships, Great Lovers maintain their attitude of openness (as we saw in the tip above), and strive to compromise. Again, if one of you insists on being right, you might as well as hang up a sign that says, "Go away. Your opinion doesn't matter." That attitude is what John Gottman so succinctly refers to as "stonewalling." If you've ever experienced it, then it's not likely you'll forget its cold, concretized surface.

36. Be Proud of Each Other.

Your public acknowledgment of how proud you are of your lover has the ability to quietly remind the world of the strength of the connection between the two of you, be it spoken or in action, in front of your partner or by someone who has observed your behavior. A lover's pride is a beacon of caring that works in the same way as a flame attracting a moth. This type of attention attracts the smiles and sweet envy of others. Now we have all seen the "displays" that masquerade as pride. This is not what I mean. I am talking about an ability these lovers have to champion their partner whether it is in the privacy of their bedroom or in a crowded restaurant. These lovers wear the nonverbal pride of their partner in their eyes. One of the more public examples of this was Nancy Reagan when she would watch the love of her life, President Reagan, giving a speech. The press corps referred to it as "The Look." Her adoration and pride in her man was apparent to all who witnessed it; yet it only mattered to her that such an exchange was felt by him. And he always understood. Pride in this case is a lovely, insulating blanket, not the avaricious trait we have been raised to think of it as.

37. Never Think of Love As Work.

You likely already have a number of to-do lists in your life. Your sex life should not be one of those lists. Your sex life is just that—about life. It is not about work, it is a privilege. We North Americans have a rather wacky way of blending work into everything we do: We eat at our desks, we network at the gym, we return calls as we walk the dog. This attitude of multi-tasking has unfortunately seeped into the bedroom. Take a tip from the Europeans: Have the attitude that both dining and sex are far too important to be done in any other way than as singular events to be relished without distraction. So the only list you should be placing your sex life on is a priority list.

38. Remember That the Way You Treat Him or Her at 8 A.M. Impacts the Way He or She Treats You at 8 P.M.

Be aware that what you say and do will always have an impact on your mate. If it's 7 A.M., and the two of you are racing around the bedroom in a mad rush to get out the door or feed the kids and get them to school, and one of you snaps at the other, that verbal quip will resonate throughout the day and into the evening. Tom and Mary always speak about themselves as "a really close couple." "We're lucky," they insist. "We've been together for fifteen years, but we're still jamming in the bedroom!" When I asked them how they keep their relationship on such an even keel, but still keep the sparks flying, they responded, "We are very careful about how we treat each other. Even if we're in bad moods, we don't take it out on the other person." Face it, we all get frantic, feel overwhelmed, and get crabby. Who can stay in a good mood all the time? But should how you're feeling inside affect how you treat your mate? Absolutely not. However, we humans sometimes forget our best intentions in times of high stress. You need to take responsibility for your behavior and not take out stress—or any other negative feeling—on your partner. So if you want to be intimate at night, you better keep that intention in mind. It's especially important to keep in mind the connection between what you say now and what you want later. If tonight is the night for a bit of wine, candlelight, and undressing, do you want to harp on each other for forgetting to do something? If you'd like to be intimate with your partner, be considerate of your partner. Actions speak volumes and you need to connect your intention with your behavior at all times. If you rush out of the house without saying good-bye, why should you expect him to be waiting for you with open arms and sex at the end of a long day? The reverse, of course, is also true: If you cuddle in bed before getting up to start the day, if you kiss him on the back of the neck as you head out the door, you are not only planting a kiss, you're planting the seed for wonderful intimacy! As Marie shared with me, "Tony and I have a five-minute morning ritual: We snuggle in bed before we get up—even our cat gets in on it, wedging himself in-between us! We both take that snuggle out the door with us." Taking the time to treat each other with care, consideration, and closeness every morning, lays the path for the evening: an evening that might move from cuddling to something a lot steamier.

39. Protect What Is Yours.

Be aware that if you find your lover attractive, so will others. Now I am assuming you are aware the majority of people have eyes and they use them on a regular basis, so if you found your honey appealing, chances are there are others who think you have great taste and know that you are one of the lucky ones. You will remain one of the lucky ones as long as you do not become complacent. I'm not advocating jealous behavior here; what I am saying is that when you were first together, chances are you weren't blasé about letting him or her know that you found that person more than desirable. You need to keep that attitude alive and kicking in your relationship—forever. So be aware that if you find your lover attractive, so will others.

40. Health Benefits of Frequent Sex.

Did you know of the many benefits of having sex with your partner? Are you aware of how frequent or regular sex enhances the overall health of your body? Consider these physiological benefits of regular sexual activity:

- enhances your immune system

- heightens mental acuity

- burns calories

- tones muscles

- strengthens the cardiovascular system

- fine tunes your metabolism

- decreases the aging factors

(Sources include: Dr. Paul Pearsall's *Superimmunity* and Dr. David Weeks's *Secrets of the Super Young.*)

41. Great Lover Moment: "She Rejuvenates Me."

A European physician in his fifties made this comment about his mid-forties fiancée: "It is as if our sex gives me more life. The only way I can describe her effect on me is to say she rejuvenates me. I feel again like I am eighteen." Having recently gone through an unpleasant divorce, he was stunned to find love again. But it was the intensity of the sexual aspect of this newfound relationship that made him decide that "This woman is who I want to have breakfast with every day. She is too important to my heart and my sex to have her get away." My point? I have two. First, that sex can be found and refound throughout one's life, so never shut the door on the potential to find someone with whom you can experience true love and true sex. And second, that sex is rejuvenating—in mind, spirit, and body.

42. Lust's Triumvirate.

Why do you need to consciously develop a desire for sex? Because you can. Because without consciously doing so, you can lose touch with the ultimate source of your lustful desires. So what is the surest way to spark your ebbing lust factor or strengthen an already-strong lust factor? By staying in touch with yourself as a sexual being. Do you ever feel like you're all head? Or you've becomes obsessed with your body—how it looks, how thin, how overweight, etc.? It's easy to become distracted in our oh-so-busy lives and become disenchanted with our bodies. And a direct result of that disenchantment is to cut ourselves off from our own sexuality. In order to stay in touch with our sexuality, we have to love our bodies. Loving our bodies means taking care of our bodies, accepting our bodies, and relishing how our bodies feel. Lust is a natural by-product of this triumvirate of the body.

43. Build a Stone House.

We've all heard the cliché that a solid house is one built on a strong foundation. Isn't this the lesson learned (too late) by the Three Little Pigs? Now seriously, ladies and gentlemen, you are in a relationship, you are already committed, and you believe in its future. Are you sure you have laid the groundwork to maintain its unwavering strength in times of stress or crisis? In my opinion, we must always err on the side of safety; here's how to shore the foundation of your relationship:

- Regularly review your romantic history together; few things add more mortar to the mix than recreating the memories that set your relationship's foundation. Trade favorite moments and share points of discovery.

- Reinforce your love and support for each other with symbols— whether it is something wacky or traditional. Does your partner like gardening tools? Photos assembled in a leather-bound album? What about a quote that describes your love for him or her?

- Have your lover tell you his or her favorite story of how you fell in love or when you first really saw that person.

The important point of this tip is to communicate and reinforce how important the relationship is to you, thereby strengthening the relationship at its core.

44. Accept That Some Problems Can't Be Solved.

Just as there are always differences in opinion in any relationship, so there are problems that won't seem to go away. And while I am a huge proponent of trying to work out any problems in a relationship using the tools of compromise to come to happy resolutions, I also know that some problems cannot be solved. In short, you can never control someone's behavior, nor can you control the people in their lives—such as a contentious relative, whether it's your mother- or father-in-law, your stepchild, or your lover's sister. So when someone or something outside of the two of you is causing a problem, you have a choice: You can either stay on your respective sides of the fence, or you can work together as a couple on the same side of the fence, so as not to let the problem divide you. Letitia had spent three years "allowing my mother-in-law to make me crazy, and it always showed up in the bedroom." But after getting some counseling, Letitia explained, "My husband and I finally resolved the issue. We agreed on certain limits to how much time his mother can spend with us. Immediately, we saw a difference in our sex life. The change was not so much from putting up better boundaries with his mother, but because my husband and I became a united front. As I say to my husband, 'She's no longer standing outside our bedroom door.'" Great Lovers have the attitude that a truly satisfying sex life does not depend on the absence of problems, but your ability to handle the problems. So you can focus on what you don't like, or begin to focus on the positive—knowing what you can change, and accepting, with grace, that which you can't change.

45. Beyond Orgasms.

It's easy—in our performance-oriented culture—to believe the myth that orgasm is the goal of sex, and that having sex is about achieving orgasms. And while all of us love the wonderful release and sensations of an orgasm, we can miss out on tremendous potential for sexual pleasure when we focus too much on bringing ourselves or our lover to orgasm. So the next time you and your lover begin playing around, make a point of delaying or even resisting orgasm. As you treat yourselves to passionate touching, oral pleasures, or the fun that toys can bring, linger. Let yourselves truly enjoy the sensations, letting them develop and come to powerful fruition, or not at all—it's your choice. By removing orgasm as a goal, you give yourself the ability to develop a keener sensitivity to all of your sexual experience. And with the increased build up, should you let yourself release into orgasm, invariably it will be to expanded levels.

46. Always Be a Beginner.

One of the attitudes most dear to a Great Lover's heart is that of always being a beginner. Related to my tip about giving yourselves permission to *not* know about sex, this tip is directed at those of you who feel pressure to become instant experts—in the arena of relationship behavior, sex techniques, or simply relating to your lover in an intimate way. One particular woman comes to mind. Sandy came to one of my seminars after her marriage of twenty-seven years had just ended. Midway through the seminar, she demurely raised her hand and confessed, "Even though I was married for such a long time, I feel like such a beginner." When I asked her what she meant, she explained that when she got married she was a virgin. She also explained that as her marriage had been coming apart for years, she and her now ex-husband had barely had sex. "I don't know anything. I feel like I'm still a virgin," she remarked in embarrassment. My response to her was immediate: "My dear, you may not know it, but you are in one of the best places to be when it comes to sex. Yes, you are a beginner, and beginners are not expected to know. You are learning and exploring. And chances are, your next man will be thrilled to know you have had only one other partner. And even if you aren't technically a true beginner, you are in a great position to assume the attitude of one: an attitude of openness and curiosity." Nothing ensures that you will have an open, exploratory attitude toward sex than if you think there is always more to know.

47. Live in a Culture of Appreciation.

We live in the most consumer-based society in the world, so it makes sense that many of us—out of sheer force of cultural programming— tend to look at relationships in the same way we are marketed to about all the products we "need" to buy. We are constantly being bombarded by commercials—on television, radio, and even our home phones—

about the next bigger, better thing. One of the effects of all this unso-licited information is that we end up feeling like we are always needing something, and end up looking at what's missing from our lives, rather than what we already have. This is a culture that tells us to measure our self-worth on extrinsic values (the house, the neighborhood, the job, the jewels, and so on); it is also a culture that suggests we should mea-sure our partners based upon what they have or can do for us, as if the qualities and characteristics of a person are concrete, attainable assets. This premise has an important corollary: often people tend to look at their partners based on what's not there (the negative), instead of what is there (the positive).

A case in point: Kane and Elizabeth are known amongst their friends as having one of the more solid and affectionate relationships. Not that they are PDA (Public Displays of Affection) specialists, but their friends know these two are still genuinely affectionate after thirty-plus years together—despite many rough patches in their marriage. From the death of their first son to both her parents dying suddenly, to the chronic illness of their child, to Kane being unemployed for years, they have clearly had their share of trials. And given this environment one would have expected their marriage to unravel or at least have some seriously frayed edges. Yet it doesn't. Why not? When I asked them how they manage their marriage and keep their sex life going, Elizabeth said simply, "I genuinely appreciate who Kane is, and believe me, I don't wear rose-colored glasses. I see him clearly for who he is, warts and all. In the beginning of our relationship, I made a decision: I chose to do what my mother had not done and look at what worked in my relation-ship rather than make myself crazy looking at what didn't work. I could have just as easily focused on what he does that I hate, but I chose in-stead to look at what I liked, loved, and appreciated about him. By be-ing able to focus on his positive qualities, I was able to get through the rough patches more easily. I knew he was doing all he could, small though that may have been." Great Lovers keep their attention on ap-preciating the other person for who he or she is—not on who they might want them to be—and accepting the reality of their relationship. Great Lovers base their relationships on what is before them: their lover, mate, or partner, who they know and love and appreciate—foibles and all. The Great Lover grows to appreciate and value his partner for who she is, not who he wants her to be. Focusing on what's missing from your partner promotes a culture of dissatisfaction, which in turn breeds a lack of contentment and an attitude that the grass is always greener. On the other hand, when a couple lives in a culture of appreciation, they reinforce an attitude of loving acceptance of each other, which in turn gives a relationship reassurance and their sex life an underlining of wonderful safety. As one sixty-five-year-old man said, "Whenever I want to start looking for greener pastures, I just start watering my own lawn."

48. Nurture Those Values You Have in Common.

Great Lovers seek out partners with values in common. Whatever these values may be, Great Lovers know that they must nurture and support these values because these beliefs are the foundation of their attraction to each other and pivotal reasons for seeking and choosing each other. Whether these values are moral, spiritual, have to do with lifestyle or a preference for flannel cotton sheets, the fact that the two of you share beliefs and attitudes in common creates a binding tie that supports and reinforces your relationship as a whole. By nurturing those values you have in common, you strengthen the underlying commitment of your relationship, from which everything else follows. That commonality is your most fertile soil and makes the relationship and its future more cohesive, stronger, and expansive. The following are four types of values that couples can develop, share, and nurture.

49. Nurture Those Values Related to Family.

One of the ways that couples can nurture their common values is through family. By family I mean both the attitude and state of mind of your household, as well as the day-to-day traditions of past, present, and future all blended into one. When you as a couple understand the differing styles of your respective birth families, then it becomes much easier to define how you want your own family to be.

Caroline and Allen met as young executives, and from early on, they knew they both wanted to have a large family: They both wanted to have children to create a legacy. Caroline was one of six children and knew intimately the joys and insanities of a large family. Allen's family was different but no less powerful: His entire extended family consisted of four, him, his sister, and his parents. Both his parents' families had perished in World War II concentration camps. Though they came from markedly different family environments, Caroline and Allen shared the common goal of creating and nurturing a family together. But this shared value also affected their sex life: "Allen, as the man in my life and in my bed, is someone I can't get enough of. All I can say is thank goodness we didn't get married any younger or we would have ten children by now!" Great Lovers like Caroline and Allen know that the fact that they both wanted and enjoy their growing family means they strengthen their love and ties to each other. If both of you aspire to have a family, already have children, or consider the two of you your complete family, nurture this connection between the two of you. By doing so, you create an entity outside of yourself, reinforcing your own relationship.

50. Nurture Those Values Related to Your Spiritual Life.

Whether we call it spiritual, religious—organized or personal—the values surrounding the internal force called "faith" has given many couples a foundation that helps them weather storms and brings great happiness and peace, not to mention an added dimension to their sex lives. This is true wherever you may find yourself on the spiritual continuum: whether you are Christian, Jewish, Muslim, or Mormon; whether you believe in God, the Goddess, or the Spirit. Sharing a sense of spirituality with your partner strengthens from within. For many couples, their shared spirituality is obvious and blatant early on in their relationship, marked by a religious ceremony of marriage. From that point on, going to Mass, a synagogue, a church, or a mosque is a regular part of their lives, one that they consciously pass down to their children. Other couples whose spiritual lives are more subtle or individual, tend to wait until they cross certain thresholds, such as becoming parents or entering a new phase in life as they age and mature. As one woman, Marian, said, "My husband and I both considered our faith background pretty immaterial until we reached our forties and sat down and asked each other, 'Where do we go from here?' We both were wanting more from life, more than our careers or other interests could answer. Then we realized that we both had similar spiritual values—a belief and desire to be kind, to be generous, to give back. These values had always been there in our lives, but we made them a more conscious part of our relationship. Our spiritual faith keeps us on the path during the day, and at night, it is a gift we give to each other." Those couples who develop a spiritual center in their relationship, and share in its power to support and heal, often find an added dimension in their relationship, one that strengthens them individually and as a couple.

51. Nurture Those Values Related to Work.

Couples who share the same work ethic; who find equal or similar pleasure and satisfaction in their work; who know where work falls in their priorities (and when it's time to take a vacation), have a much easier time navigating through life. For most of us, work is essential—be it working for a salary or handling the day-to-day work of raising children. So while we may all define work differently, how we approach work, and where it figures in our list of priorities, is what matters most in relationships. If one of you, for instance, loves his or her work but has trouble leaving it at the office, and the other person only works to pay his or her bills, then this difference in attitude can cause conflict. As one client, Jim, told me, "Carmen and I used to fight all the time because I felt she was a workaholic. She had no time for me. But it wasn't until I said those words out loud—'You don't have time for me'—that she was finally able to hear what I had been trying to tell her. She had become validated by the fact that she could do so much, so she kept looking for more to do. Work and being busy had become her life. After she finally listened to how her work was affecting me, we sat down and made a timetable to try to blend our work and personal needs. We ultimately wrestled the issue to the ground. Needless to say, after having clarified what our work values are, we now create more time for just the two of us. And it has made all the difference." When the two of you agree on the importance and value of work, then this shared attitude will make it easier to agree on how you allocate and prioritize your time. You can decide ahead of time to work a certain percentage of the day or week; to commit two hours every second day for leisure; and three nights a week at home—for sex or simple relaxation.

52. Nurture Those Values Related to Money.

Money is often the third dimension of your relationship. When you and your lover share similar values about money, how to spend it, how to save it, and how to play with it, you quite simply make life smoother. Also, there is often an unspoken power dynamic set up by the person who brings in the most money, and addressing that dynamic is often as difficult a conversation to have as who is more in love with whom. Another complicating factor is that people can speak and think so differently about money, that even if you are discussing the money problems in your relationship, you can't assume you're talking about the same thing. One couple comes to mind.

Margaret and Ted looked like a young, successful, childless couple—from the outside. On the inside, there was mounting tension and frustration. Ted was a successful Wall Street executive who, by all accounts, made a lot of money. Their value system about money changed when

Margaret, a former research executive, returned to university to do graduate work. When Margaret stopped bringing in money, tension began to build between her and Ted—so much so that they stopped having sex. It wasn't until Margaret said, "If you think you're the only opinion that counts because you're the only one earning, we have a big problem. Quite frankly I think you'll be very happy by yourself with your money because I am ready to walk." Together, they realized that after ten years of being together, they had to re-create the money values in their marriage. They had to review what money meant to each of them, what they expected from it, and how they wanted to spend it. As soon as they processed these thoughts about money, the tension between them disappeared—as if overnight. It's crucial that each of you be clear about how money be treated in your relationship and in your life—so money doesn't come between you in your bedroom.

53. Court Your Lover, Forever.

Courting your lover is as much a behavior as it is an attitude. In distant eras, the essence of courtly love was putting forth the idea that the person you love is the chosen *one*. And although some of this attitude still exists today, many of us get a little lethargic once we are into the relationship. When we first fall in love and get together as a couple, we tend to treat each other with kid gloves. We do so because we're not so sure how this new person will react to us, so we tend to be more careful, more delicate, more solicitous. In the getting-to-know-you-better stage, we also discover many things that tickle our partner's sense of humor, touch his or her heart, and generally have that lover give us insider awareness of what makes him or her feel special. One of the most impactful ways we show a partner's specialness is by delivering our attention in ways that reveal how he or she is our focus, and that our lover's opinion matters. But as relationships grow, and as we become more used to each other, some of this focused energy dwindles. Great Lovers know that by maintaining the focused energy of courtship throughout their lives, they ensure not only that the initial romantic spirit stays true, but that their lovers will always feel special, never taken for granted. So I recommend taking a tip from those knights and ladies of old. There are two main ways you can keep the courting spirit alive: first, remember that a large part of courting is in taking the time to present ourselves in a physically appealing way. Chances are you used to spend more time dressing when you were dating; resume this attention to detail and maintain it throughout your relationship. Second, continue making the courting gestures that seemed so effortless and exciting when the two of you were falling in love. Here are some suggestions:

- bring your lover a bag of juicy Concord grapes for lunch

- pick out several romantic classics from the video store and suggest a movie-marathon weekend

- gentlemen, offer your hand when she alights from a cab

- ladies, make him his favorite cookies—for breakfast—and deliver them to bed with his coffee

There is tremendous power in courting, and Great Lovers revisit its potency regularly.

54. Je Ne Sais Quoi—or "I Just Can't Explain It."

Great Lovers know they have a special something, a chemistry and attraction factor that their partner feels on a cellular level, but to a large degree defies description. This indescribable feeling is the "*je ne sais quoi*" of appeal. I often hear the same conversation between lovers: "There is just something about you." Neither person cares to define it; both partners are just thrilled they've got that whatever-it-is. As countless seminar attendees have shared, the appeal and attraction of their lover is not about idealized looks. It's about that special appeal factor that is uniquely yours. So my tip is this: Sometimes it's best to accept that you cannot define why you and your lover are attracted to each other or love each other. In allowing this quality to go undefined, you give your relationship an aura of mystery, which in turn breathes romance and sexual heat into your relationship.

55. Seasonal Sex.

Change is a natural and predictable part of our lives, and in the same way that we expect seasonal variations to renew and refresh us, we need to allow changes in our sexual lives to rejuvenate us and our relationships. So for those of you who feel that sexually things between you have become too routine or by the book, I have come up with a game I call "Seasonal Sex." The idea came from a couple who shared the story that every summer they stopped having intercourse, due to the lack of air conditioning at their family beach house. "It was too damn sticky," one of them remarked, so they chose to satisfy each other orally during beach weekends. By the end of that first summer, they had a new name for it—"Summer Sex." The following spring, when they began trying to get pregnant, they used a deep, penetrating position, which as you may guess, they called "Spring Sex." To take this tip home with you, so to speak, the only rule you have to remember is to create your preferred positions for each season. One woman had this to say, "Not only did this have us look at what our favorite positions are, but it gave us shorthand to use in public when we wanted to let each other know what was on our minds." One example: "I look forward to seeing your friends this summer." Translation? "I want to suck on the twins (i.e. his testicles). Now we have added our own important calendar days to expand our repertoire. Thanksgiving sex is a big favorite."

56. Timetables Are for Trains.

This tip has to do with not getting stuck on a timetable for sex. I realize this may seem to contradict the tip above, but au contraire, not so.

What I am referring to here is the tendency to have sex once a week on Sunday morning, at 7:30 A.M., because that is when the kids are watching cartoons and you have approximately twenty minutes during *Spongebob SquarePants*. For the majority of people, if their sex becomes so same-same that they know all the moves and triggers, they tune out and start to avoid it. Now, knowing your opportunities is crucial for parents and any busy couple best err on the side of flexibility, for you wouldn't want to waste a presented opportunity simply because it wasn't scheduled. New parents Tara and James take advantage of those opportunities with "What we call 'Sex Lite.' It is a few minutes in which we have actual intercourse and connect physically, but know ahead of time that we don't have time to go to the end. Initially I thought it would make me frustrated and instead I leave with the feel of him inside of me, knowing more is yet to come."

57. Enlarge Your Expectations—for Yourself, Your Lover, and Your Relationship.

As Mark Twain said, "Even if you are on the right track, if you stand still, the train will run you over." Great Lovers do not remain static about their expectations of relationships, or each other. They continue to see the "us" of a relationship as a growing dynamic event, and they expect to see concrete returns on what they put into it. This tip also incorporates how you approach life in general: Do you see yourself and the world around you through a glass that is half full or half empty? When your glass is half full, you give yourself the opportunity to always grow bigger, be bigger, and have bigger expectations. How does this attitude affect your sex life? It keeps you always looking for the new and unexpected. It keeps you believing that more is always possible. One woman, Erin, related this, "My older sister was a great role model on how to keep expanding my relationship. She said we had to constantly review what we expected from one another sexually and emotionally and to never think there is a ceiling on what is possible. And eleven years into my relationship, I can tell you, she was right on." So as you face your life together, always expect the best to happen: that the two of you will keep refinding each other in passion, love, and lust. But first, you've got to want that to happen.

58. Minimize Your Expectations—for Yourself, Your Lover, and Your Relationship.

When I say minimize your expectations, I am referring to minimizing the impact of and keeping in perspective the mediaized messages about how lovers and people in relationships should be. When couples are able to avoid the pitfall of responding to what others tell them to do or say sexually, then they avoid the "shoulda, woulda, coulda" syndrome. We are all so inundated by messages and expectations that it's very difficult to ignore them. But to borrow from the ideas of many philosophies, when you listen to what's "out there" instead of what's "in here," you automatically disrupt your connection with the here and now. You are no longer in the moment, but instead constantly thinking of how and what you should be doing, rather than doing it. However, when you believe you are trying your best, then you allow yourself to enjoy the pleasure that is right in front of you. And sexually speaking, this means that you are inside the moment with your lover. As Kyle shared in a seminar, "I have attended every sexual workshop you can imagine. I was always looking for some sexual Holy Grail I had yet to discover. It wasn't until I met my Buddhist wife that I understood that the reason I felt something was always missing was because I was looking outside of myself. When I shifted my focus to what I was already enjoying sexually, I realized I had been belittling my own experiences, which were and are pretty fabulous." When lovers learn to accept themselves, and their sexual experience, at face value, they tend to experience a deeper level of sexual satisfaction.

59. *Let Passion and Sex Be a Reward for You As a Couple, Not a Chore or Obligation.*

And how delightful you can reward yourselves as generously and as often as you'd like—your only limit is your imagination. If one feels that lovemaking is a chore or an obligation, then you need a new dictionary, a new partner, or a new attitude. This is normally an issue when there is disparate sexual natures between the two parties. Merritt and Thomas decided to take a tip from their children: Just as the couple had given their kids treats for good behavior, so they deserved a reward system for their sex life as a way to move out of the humdrums. "We not only moved out of the humdrums, we expanded our fantasy play. We each have a mental list of what qualifies as 'good behavior,' so if I decide Thomas was 'good' because he picked up the kids from soccer, I let him know and then he gets to request what type of reward he wants. And vice versa for me. I happen to know lemon meringue pie gets me just about everything I want."

60. *Don't Get Carried Away by Performance.*

Hmmmm. We all want to do things well, but what we need to be aware of when it comes to sex is not how the films depict couples together, but how *we* are together. Let me make this analogy between clothing and sex: You wear the clothes, your clothes don't wear you. In terms of sex, you have the sex, the sexual act is not using you. And both sexes fall prey to this pressure to perform. Women have commented, "He used six different positions in the first three minutes and I'm thinking, 'Whoa, tiger, where is the camera?'" Men have related, "She was so loud I had to put my hand over her mouth." Performance is just that, it is for show and for stage—not for lovemaking. As I suggest to couples, when you are being sexual, *focus* on the pleasure of you and your partner, not on how well you're doing a move.

61. Make Lovemaking a Conscious Lifestyle Choice.

In the same way you make lifestyle choices about where you want to live, this falls into how you want to live. This idea came from a couple who shared at a seminar that they did not want to have happen what had happened to a number of their friends after children . . . no sex. And even though they were practical enough to know their sex life would alter after they had children, they were determined to preserve their sexual connection. As the man said, "Despite how busy we both are, our sex life is too important for us to leave it to chance events. We make a time commitment to keep our bodies in shape and we do the same for our sex lives. Now we just have to be more creative. We choose having sex over not having sex any day." Great Lovers know they have to make a conscious decision to have lovemaking be part of their lifestyle, and that means making the time, creating a plan, and always following through.

62. You Are Committed 24/7.

This commitment means you need to acknowledge that you are in the relationship for the long haul and be aware of this on an hourly, daily basis. This means always acting on the intention you have for your relationship. When a couple has the intention to make it work regardless of what is going on or has happened, they have a stronger, more supportive framework from which to branch out. Hillary highlighted the flip side of this tip when she said, "When Evan and I married, I realized I had to toss my 'I can leave whenever I wish' attitude. This had been a behavior pattern I'd always relied on so I could end a relationship when I wanted. I always had one foot out the door, and needless to say, this attitude always showed up in my actions. Now, since I've finally learned what commitment means, it is both scary and intensely comforting to know Evan and I are each other's safety net." My advice here is prickled by the flip side of Hillary's story: constant awareness of your commitment to each other ensures that you will remain committed.

63. Style Differences.

Great Lovers are able to accept that each partner may have his or her own communicating style. By listening and speaking thoughtfully to each other, you can create ways to support those differences. Genny knew that even though Clark was up early in the morning, his ears didn't work until after his first coffee. She jokingly called it the Caffeine Bridge. Clark knew that the moment he raised his voice in his Mediterranean family's style of clearing the air, he had just lost Genny. Nothing in her WASPy background prepared her for those emotional outbursts. Solution? Genny realized she had to wait until Clark was post-coffee, post-shower before any conversations, and Clark saved his more excitable style of expressing himself for his birth family and adopted a new style with Genny that was calmer and smoother in delivery. So be aware of how your communicating styles may differ from each other, and take out the emotion when you are trying to be heard.

64. Be Honest and Forgiving of Your Own Human Frailties.

The human qualities we often refer to as frailties are often those we have little control over. I am speaking about the physical qualities more than social behaviors such as a bad temper or being very sensitive. When we don't like something about ourselves, it is often because someone else told us they didn't like this quality. In this tip I am advising you to know and accept your limitations so that you can be happy. Sam was always very self-conscious about his body hair; this sensitivity stemmed back to when he was younger and was constantly teased by his older sisters. When he met Leah, his current girlfriend, he got a whole new perspective on his hair. They were on the way to the pool when Leah came up behind him and kissed his shoulder. At first, he moved away and said, "Oh, you don't want to do that." Her bewildered response, "Do what?" He replied, "Kiss this," pointing to the hair on his shoulders. Leah smiled and said, "Why do you think I put my lips there? I love that soft, furry part of you." In one nanosecond, Sam no longer saw his hair as a problem.

65. Be Honest and Forgiving of Your Lover's Human Frailties.

The same holds true for how we think about our partner. Of course he or she has faults. Of course he or she is not perfect. Did you ever think that person was? No. So why spend time or mental energy on criticizing or judging your lover? Don't keep a running list of how someone bugs you. Blaine explains, "When we were first together, Gary was very concerned about my reaction to his snoring. It had been something that his ex-wife had complained about constantly, to the point that they ended up sleeping in separate rooms. It took me months before he was convinced that his snoring wasn't an issue for me. Besides, I had him sleep in a different position, more on his side, and that took care of a lot of the problem." However, when you are honest and forgiving of a person's faults, accepting your partner for who she or he is, then you give that person the gift of unconditional love, padding your bed, so to speak, with joy and the greatest potential for sexual peace.

66. Understand That All Aspects of Your Relationship Affect Your Sexual Relationship.

If you are experiencing tension or pain in your life due to work pressure (you hate your new boss), a family crisis (an older parent becomes critically ill), an individual issue (you're feeling the inevitable effects of aging), you need to expect your sex life to be affected. Once you are aware of this connection, you can then take steps not to let your sexual relationship suffer. How? There are a few things you can do. First, by your simply being aware, you have lessened the negative impact on your sex life. Second, take steps to take care of yourself in other ways, so these negative feelings do not leak or overflow into your intimate relationship with your partner. And third, try to let your sexual relationship be your haven, your succor—the thing the two of you turn to when life outside becomes hazardous.

67. Understand That Separating the Various Aspects of Your Relationship Can Put Those Parts at Risk.

Fortunately or unfortunately, this tip is directed mostly at the men in the audience. Why? Because men are more natural compartmentalizers than women. Men tend to focus exclusively on one project at a time, and women tend to exist more comfortably juggling numerous tasks and being able to focus on two or three things at once. Men tend to compartmentalize these sections of their lives: work, home, family, sex, sports, whatever. The risk of keeping things in separate areas is that your attention and energy stays in one area too long, to the detriment of the other areas. Use your car's tires as a metaphor: You need all four tires to drive safely, and need to maintain proper air pressure in all of them. However, you also need to maintain balance, balancing the attention that each compartment gets. I have met many workaholic men who are now unhappily single because the compartment holding their former wife or girlfriend never got enough focus.

68. Be Open to "Tune-Ups."

These tune-ups can be done with a professional or just the two of you, in which you and your partner review the mechanics of your relationship. I learned this tip from a couple who had been through enormous pain and suffering in their relationship, only to come out on the other side complete winners. Kim and Daniel's relationship had been in the absolute toilet when one of them (Kim) had had an affair. All trust had been broken. The anger was deep and destructive. Neither of them felt any hope that they could salvage their relationship, but they tried couple's counseling in a last-ditch effort. What they discovered was that as they began to see past their anger (not an easy thing, to be sure), they were able to get back in touch with why they first liked and grew to love each other. As Kim and Daniel began to heal the wounds on both sides, forgive each other, and renew their commitment to their relationship, they realized that one of the reasons the affair had happened in the first place was that they had lost each other in the busyness of day to day life. Starved for affection and attention, Kim had reached out to an old boyfriend—surely not the answer. However, Daniel was able to see that Kim still loved him. Now, five years later, they not only set aside time each month to nurture their love, but they also do "tune-ups" with their couples therapist whenever they feel the need to air grievances. The therapist provides additional support in a less charged atmosphere.

69. Be Willing to Challenge Your Own Sexual Comfort Zone.

This tip is a reminder for all of us who give in too easily to what feels comfortable. It's human nature, of course, to remain doing things that are comfortable and familiar, and this rule applies to sex as much as it does anything in life. But if you remain hemmed in by your sexual comfort zone, you only limit your sexual experience, and your degree of pleasure (and that of your partner). So the next time you find yourself falling into the quickest and easiest way you know to pleasure you or your partner, pause and consider changing your route. And there are plenty of ideas to play with—simply read ahead!

70. Remember That Just Because It Isn't Important to You Doesn't Mean It Isn't Important to Her.

This tip came to me when I heard about a friend who went out of town on business. She was going to be gone a week and asked her husband to water her plants. When she arrived home, she was really upset to find all of her plants dead. But the biggest reason she was upset was because her husband didn't understand what the big deal was. Bad enough her plants were dead; he didn't even care that they had mattered to her. Many couples have shared similar stories, especially around holidays such as Valentine's Day. Gentlemen, if you think this day of hearts and roses is silly, but you know it matters to her, then you need to make the day and its symbolism matter to you—even if you don't really "get it." And ladies, men too want to be romanced, so don't make the mistake of thinking that your showing up is Valentine enough. So whether you show your lover you get what he or she is into—be it a plant, a baseball cap collection, classic, first-edition books, or fuzzy dice—anytime you show your partner you know something is important to him or her, you speak volumes to that person's heart. And it is a short trip from the heart to other areas of their anatomy.

How to Be a Great Lover in Behavior

With your attitude informing all your moves, you are now prepared to put your thoughts, feelings, and desires into action—whether in the bedroom or outside of it. Since 90 percent of foreplay takes place outside of the room where most sex is initiated, you need to keep in mind that how you behave toward your partner deeply affects your sexual relationship. Great Lovers know that when they nurture their relationships, they ensure that Great Sex can happen. In this section, you will see how you can strengthen the foundation of your relationship, put more of your intentions into actions, and become the Great Lover you are destined to be.

71. Speak to Each Other As You Did When You First Met.

Many office associates witness the power of this tip firsthand when they overhear colleagues speak to their lovers. In one office I was in, there were two such couples, one about to be married, the other married 30+ years. Sue would light up like a little beam when her fiancé, Jay, called; but the really sweet thing was to see Jerry's curmudgeonly face soften as he would gently answer, "Hello, Sweetheart," when his wife, Carol, called. This secret is about continuing to spark the fires of that falling-in-love sex and carrying it through—no matter how long the two of you have been together. When you were courting him or her, and/or first seducing him or her, your intention was always: Treat your new love in a special way, and let him or her know how special he or she is to you. This intention automatically carries over into your voice. If you remind yourself of this intention, it will come across in the way you speak to her or him. I promise. Deirdre, a busy bond trader, has a policy whenever her husband calls: he is always put through. Her rationale is simple: "He is the most important man in my life, and I will always make time to speak to him."

72. *Gentlemen, Let Her Know She's Irresistible.*

Gentlemen, ladies love to be reminded of how she first turned your head, made your groin ache with desire, or made your heart swoon. Was it the gold blouse she wore on your first date? The way she wore her hair swooped up at the base of her neck? Was it the tight black skirt that hugged her derriere? If you don't remember, then start digging. Alan remembers with laser clarity "How that green linen dress hugged Cheri's caboose on our first date. And the way those hubba-hubba shoes made her legs look." Half way through the evening, he also remembers saying to himself, "This is not a dinner date. I am really into this woman. Since then (we've been together two years), I hang that green dress on the bedroom door as I leave for work whenever I want to remind her how irresistible she is." No doubt you too, have a way of letting your partner know *now* she's still irresistible to you.

73. Ladies, Let Him Know He's Irresistible.

Men *need* to know you are attracted to them. They want to feel as they did when you first got together: that he has something you can't resist and that you can't get enough of him. Tell him, and show him. Different from paying attention to him in ways outside of the bedroom, this secret has all to do with the bedroom. When he's undressing, watch him. When he steps out of the shower, watch him. Lick the droplets of water off his body simply because you can't resist. When he's ready to walk out the door, pull him to you and kiss him, deeply. Men pay attention to your actions as a way to predict whether there is sex in the future.

74. Great Lover Moment: "I Simply Can't Get Enough of Her."

A friend's father who didn't marry until he was fifty was the quintessential international bachelor, as the head of a major pharmaceutical company, he was chased by women across continents. Very aware of his father's single days, my friend knew his mother had to have had something very special to have finally captured the heart of such an incorrigible man. He went to his father asking him one question, "How did you know Mom was the one?" His father's response was immediate: "I simply couldn't get enough of her then, and I simply can't get enough of her now." My point? Use this question as your litmus test: If you still cannot get enough of your lover, you know you've met your match.

75. Take the Pulse of a Relationship on an Ongoing Basis.

Great Lovers are always aware, alert, and active. These three states of mind mean that they never assume that everything is okay in the relationship. A few years ago, Karl and Keren saved their twelve-year marriage. They had become so demoralized by the cold emptiness of their relationship, both of them had given up all hope that they could ever feel passion for each other again. At the time, Keren remembers, "We had become so complacent. We had stopped even trying to communicate or do fun things together. Karl would go to work. I would go to work. We'd go to bed each night, turning our backs on each other. It was like I was sleeping with my brother." What turned it around? One of Keren's girlfriends had suggested they come to a Sexuality Seminar for couples. Karl said, "Basically, we thought we had nothing to lose." When they heard couples having fun, and especially connecting this fun to their love and commitment, Karl and Keren began to feel a flicker of hope. "We looked at each other," Keren remembers, "and realized that we had stopped trying." Great Lovers check in with each other all the time. Weekly. Daily. Monthly. They ask each other how they feel, they make a point of knowing what's going on with the other at work, with friends, with family members. They don't assume they know all there is to know about the other. They are active in the relationship, treating it as if it were a living, breathing organism that needs food and air to grow. And by all means, don't assume nothing is happening if nothing is being said. Great Lovers are proactive. They don't accept silence without at first making sure their partner is happy. Peg and Mike learned that lesson well. In the early part of their marriage, they assumed that silence was a good thing. Until one Sunday afternoon when Peg said she was going out shopping with her girlfriends. "I can still remember the look on his face," recalls Peg. "He was practically blue he was so angry. When I asked him what was wrong, he blasted me about always ditching him on Sundays. He wanted Sundays to be about us, as a couple. I didn't know. When I asked him why he had never told me, he said defensively, 'I thought you knew.'" "I thought you knew." Does that refrain sound familiar? If so, then you need to become proactive. You need to make it a point to know what's going on inside of your partner's head and heart. When I asked Peg how she and Mike had fixed their problem, she said they never took silences for granted again. "The irony is, I was totally flattered that he wanted to spend Sunday with me—I had assumed he liked watching sports on TV. From that point on, we made a point of telling each other what we wanted to do on the weekends. We didn't always want to do the same thing, but we never made the mistake of not knowing." If you don't check in with each other on a regular basis, you will lose the pulse of the relationship and risk losing your connection to your partner. Great Lovers take the pulse of the relationship on an ongoing basis. They ask questions, they offer ideas. They stay active, alert, and aware, and treat their relationship as a living organism. That, they say, is the key to keeping the heart of a relationship pumping with life, with each partner feeling connected and cared for.

76. Ladies, Acknowledge the Things He Does for You.

Men tend to show their love through their actions, so don't take them for granted. I realize this may sound very simplistic, but bear in mind that he can't know he has done something you appreciate unless you tell him. As comedian Sam Kinison said, "Ladies, let him know when he's done it well!" And don't overlook all the other things he does well either. We often are very unaware of the pride our men take in their "manly jobs" such as edging the flower bed, their snow removing finesse, and taking your car in for servicing. These are things they do with you in mind—your pleasure at looking at the garden, your ease getting out of the driveway, your safety in the car. As one mother of three put it, "I always praise Dean and let him know he has done a good job. It's directly related to our great sex. I know if he doesn't feel appreciated I don't get appreciated, and I love sex too much for that." So ladies, let him know that by virtue of his actions, he has made your life better.

77. Gentlemen, Pay Deep Attention to Her— in Whatever Way She Wants.

Remember that in order to seduce her body, you must seduce her mind. And the absolute, number-one fastest and best way to seduce her mind is by paying deep and real attention to her. Women love this. Trust me when I tell you they thrive on it and will pay you back in spades! Women need to feel safe, connected, and relaxed in order to open themselves up to a man. The reality is that there is hardly a greater turn-on for women than knowing they are being listened to and truly understood. It is a tried-and-true equation: pay deep attention to your lover's wants, needs, thoughts, and feelings, and you have tapped into one of the greatest seduction secrets of all time. If you need proof, just watch any movie, and in this case movies tend to reflect real life: even the most nebbishy guy gets the girl in the end. Why? Because he figures out that if he really tuned in to what she wants and needs, and he came through, then he'll get the girl in the end. A case in point is Bill Murray's buffoon character in *Groundhog Day,* who in the end won Andie MacDowell's heart.

But after the honeymoon, many men tend to forget this valuable connection, and lose sight of how important it is to keep paying attention to her. And I'm not just speaking of paying attention to a woman's needs during lovemaking—that goes without saying. I'm talking about paying deep attention to your lover's wants and needs outside the bedroom as well. This is absolutely key to keeping your sex life sizzling in perpetuity. The tricky part can be learning the best ways to pay attention so you hit the mark. Attention can be anything from how you listen (often the most crucial), to showing that you really *know* her, *care* about her, *understand* her, and that you've taken the time to translate that knowledge into action. So listen to her. Listen when she tells you what she is feeling, and respond in kind. Listen when she tells you about her childhood memories, or about the argument she had with her boss, or about what movies, wine, songs, places she loves. Listen to everything she is saying, both out loud and through actions, in the same way you did when you first met and she was the most important thing in the world to you. The more in tune you are with what matters to her, the more you will know what to do in order to seduce her, body and mind. Here is a collection of a few thoughtful and seductive suggestions gathered from my more outspoken clients. Some or all of these may inspire you, but take notice: Whatever you choose to do, however you decide to pay deep attention to your lover, your action must carry the weight of your intention. In other words, what you do and how you do it will have an impact only if it shows that you know what makes *her* happy. Robert's plan of a weekend hiking sojourn will not work for a woman who treasures her Sunday mornings at home, just as a beautiful floral arrangement will not have the desired effect when sent to a woman who has severe allergies. Remember, this is all about paying attention to your individual lady and coming through with attentions that are particularly meaningful to her:

- If her parents are coming to town for a visit and you know this stresses her out, do something to help her out. Book her a massage for the afternoon before they arrive, or act as the buffer if the familiar family argument starts to erupt. It will mean a lot to her to know you are on her side.

- The next time she wears an outfit that you like, even if you've seen it before, notice her in it, and then tell her how beautiful she looks in it. Repeat behavior as needed.

- If you know she is having a difficult week at work, send her a thoughtful gift—whatever is special to her (one gentleman, whose lady loves *The Wizard of Oz*, sent her a pair of red, satin, bedroom slippers with a note reading, "click three times and imagine it's Friday"). I know this may sound a tad predictable, but I also know it works. Women just melt when they receive a gift from their lovers. You will have just made her week a whole lot better, and all her friends envious.

- Notice when she is feeling overwhelmed and offer to assist her. Sometimes that might mean doing an errand for her, other times it could mean taking over her responsibilities in the house for the evening and sending her off to take a guilt-free bubble bath.

- If she tells you she doesn't enjoy spending time with certain people, do your best to limit those interactions. One gentleman, whose wife found a colleague of his particularly distasteful, politely but continually declined invitations to double-date. Forcing a woman to be around people she despises is a sure way to roll up the sexual red carpet.

- Rent the movie she has been wanting to see (even if you've seen it), pick up the red wine she favors (even if you'd prefer a beer), get her the new CD by her favorite recording artist (even if you think he is terrible), pick up the low-fat frozen yogurt she likes on your way home (even if you want ice cream).

It's the little gestures that add up. Never forget that giving your partner your attention is one of the most seductive things you can do. And be aware, gentlemen, women often say the most important things the most softly—in an almost wistful way. It is often your attention in some sweet, unexpected way that will have them fall in love with you on a daily basis. And that, my friends, is a very good thing.

78. Act Quickly to Spot and Fix a Problem.

No relationship is without its storms. Problems, conflicts, and challenges always surface—after all, this is real life we're talking about. But Great Lovers act quickly to spot and fix a problem. This quality is related to their knack for taking the pulse of the relationship on a regular basis. If you both are present in the relationship, you will naturally be aware of what's going on with each other, as well as within yourself. Glen and Gary were roommates in college so when Glen moved to the town in which Gary and Carla live, they welcomed him into their social circle. The problems started when Glen seemed to invite himself on all their dates. Carla was patient at first, but after a few months of dating "two men," she was becoming frustrated and angry—at both Gary, her boyfriend of three years, and Glen, who she was beginning to think of as "the interloper." She also wanted Gary to correct the problem on his own. Carla felt it was "his duty" to know that Glen shouldn't always be invited on their dates, so she didn't say anything. A few more months went by until one weekend, Carla just blew up. "I couldn't stand it anymore, and I really got mad. I was about to break up with Gary!" She finally got Gary's attention. Gary completely responded to Carla's feelings, acknowledging how he had let Glen come between them. But a lot of Carla's frustration and pain could have been avoided if she had only said something to Gary sooner. Great Lovers know that problems and conflicts are a normal part of life and relationships, so they learn how to spot a problem and fix it quickly—with compassion and the confidence that they will find a solution. They take responsibility for anything that affects or impacts their relationship—no matter who is to blame or what is the cause. If you approach a problem with this attitude, you will more than likely find a resolution. So next time something comes up, choose a good moment, think about what you want to say, and share your feelings with your partner. Nine times out of ten, your partner will be able to hear you right away.

79. Learn from Your Mistakes.

In short, learn from your mistakes. Most of us have had at least one previous relationship that we can look back on and realize things we might have done differently. Even if he left you. Even if she was the reason you broke up. A relationship always takes two, which means that both of you contributed to a relationship's not working out. Sometimes relationships end naturally, with both parties realizing more or less simultaneously that the relationship is not satisfying enough, not challenging enough, not enough—period. However, whenever relationships end, it's up to you to put them behind you so that you can be completely involved in your current relationship. But that does not mean you should repeat your mistakes. In other words, learn from your mistakes. Gentlemen, I'm afraid this piece of advice is mostly for you. Women seem to have an easier time making sense of relationships that did not work and making sure they don't make the same mistakes twice. Men, unfortunately, tend to forget. Or not even bother to examine what went wrong to begin with. But let me say this first: all of us make mistakes, and none of us is perfect. We all have annoying habits, insecurities, or moments of indifference—all of which have the potential to drive our partner crazy, push him or her away from us, or make that person feel bad. If you are in a relationship and you want it to work, then it's absolutely vital that you be honest about your particular weak areas so that you don't let the new relationship take on any negative baggage that has no reason being around in the first place. What really bugged your past partner? If you're now in your first relationship, what have friends or family consistently remarked upon about you that makes them uncomfortable or hurt? It is not fun to look at our least admirable traits, but when you know them, you can address them. When I asked a gentleman why his last relationship suddenly ended, he replied, "She said she didn't want to be a golf widow." I asked him, "Isn't that why your marriage didn't work out? Hadn't Kathy complained that you spent all your free time on the golf course and not enough time together?" He looked at me in surprise, "Yes." And then you could see the sadness creep into his face. "I really tried to make the relationship work. I guess I was just too set in my ways." In the common-sense category of recommendations, I suggested his next woman be a person who golfed. All of us can be set in our ways; it happens quite naturally as we age—and there's no avoiding that—but we can avoid certain behaviors that are destined to alienate or hurt or disappoint our partners. So what does this tip boil down to? You need to incorporate your past experiences into your present relationship in a positive way.

80. Be an Explorer.

In the attitude section, you learned how important it is to develop an open mindset about all things sexual. In this section, we are focused on your behavior—especially when it comes to how your relationship affects your sex life. So how do you not only become an explorer in attitude, but one in behavior as well? You keep each other on your toes. You inspire each other to do new things. You encourage each other to try new ways of being together. What do I mean? Let me give you a few examples.

- If you're homebody types, used to spending your weekends cuddled up at home watching movies on the DVD, then plan a weekend around outdoor adventures—a simple walk through the woods can do wonders to refresh you.

- If you're a couple who is used to splitting up on the weekends, he's raking leaves, she's doing errands, or vice versa—then change your routine: either rake the leaves together or do your errands together. The point is: do whatever it is together.

- If you're a couple who already loves spending time alone, perhaps now is the time to plan a small dinner party—be it at your home or hosted at a restaurant. Consider serving an aphrodisiac menu—you need not tell your guests until afterward.

All of these suggestions are meant to break up your set routine and give the two of you a new way of spending time together. The more time you spend together having fun, the more you get in touch with your enjoyment of each other. And that enjoyment directly impacts your degree of sexual intimacy.

81. No Psychic Sex.

You cannot expect your lover to read your mind. I will tell you that lovers who have taken the risk and shared what they knew have reaped huge rewards in the intimacy department. Now I realize that this is often easier said than done because we don't want to be judged or put our feelings at risk. But it's important to be honest and ask for what you want. If you're uncomfortable doing this, rather than bringing up the subject of what you might want to try in daylight, have the talk while horizontal with low lighting and snuggling, not while in mid-activity.

This way you can feel secure, not be interrupted, and while holding each other, you can feel your lover's unspoken physical reactions to comments that will guide you to expand or shift the topic slightly.

Take this example. Carrie wanted to have more anal sex. She adored it, and with Marcus she had never tried it. The first time she broached the subject, they were snuggling on the couch watching a porn film and that act came on. She said she knew she'd like to try it. She phrased it in such a way as to not offend Marcus and so he was comfortable obliging. By saying, "I want to know about this," he didn't need to be reminded of when and where Carrie had tried anal sex before him. At the same time, when you do share requests or desires, you need to be specific; everyone needs details and directions in order to be effective. If he or she has just hit a hot spot, reinforce their action with a "Oh, do that again." Or "I love when you play with my lips like that." Keep in mind this minor caveat: It's always best to avoid revealing that the source of your request may be others you may have done this with in the past. In the gentlest way, always try to share what you want to know sexually with your partner.

82. Seal Your Lips.

For both sexes your relationship is a very private experience and the last thing Great Lovers want is others to hear a Tommy Lee and Pamela description of their lovemaking. There probably isn't a bigger nightmare for most men than if their woman shares intimate details with others. Why? Because they don't want to be given a mental image of the things they do sexually with their partner. However, women in general talk more openly about their sex lives and not from a prurient, "Yeah, baby, I'm so hot in bed" attitude. Rather, it's a mostly innocent kind of cultural information-sharing women do. But it's always best to be private about your relationship. There is an unspoken power that accompanies discretion and Great Lovers know this power intimately: When it comes to personal disclosure, they tend to err on the side of less is more. This tip, therefore, is quite simple: be private. Similar to that cliché about how those with old money never have to talk about their money, this tip taps into the strength a couple can gain from letting the most intimate details of their lives remain between them—whether the subject at hand is money, their emotional life, or sex. The irony is that everyone will know your sex life is strong because you don't talk about it. So restrict discussions of your relationship with anyone other than those involved: the two of you and your most intimate family and friends. All of us want to feel good about what we do and who we are with, but we do not need to "spread the word" of this most personal side of ourselves indiscriminately. However, I do not mean to imply that you should be evasive or aloof. Au contraire; answer any inquiries about your personal life in honest, but general terms: "He is a most pleasurable lover." "We connect well." "She rocks my world." Great Lovers know their nondisclosure isn't about secrecy; it is about something more special—their intimacy.

83. Don't Compare Yourselves to Anyone, Much Less Hollywood Idols.

To be a Great Lover, you need to possess a strong degree of comfort with your own unique appeal and look. I am only too aware of this as I am an identical twin. Although we look very similar to each other, we have always possessed a special unique appeal that is absolutely distinct. From the time I was a little unit, my sister and I have never attracted the same boys or men, nor have we been attracted to the same men. This uniqueness and our awareness and acceptance of it has not only empowered us in our respective relationships, it has also shored up our confidence in ourselves. You need to keep in mind that the so-called natural look of Hollywood idols is the carefully crafted result of behind-the-scenes maneuvering by an army of great wardrobe stylists, makeup artists, photographers, and airbrushing. Throw in the legacy of strong genes, and the Hollywood stars can't help but look fantastic—all of the time. The job of stars is just that: to act in front of a camera and look good. Need I mention the ubiquitous digital retouching of models' breasts in fashion shoots and body parts in porn images? Further, remember that the depictions of love, sex, and intimacy on the big and little screens are fabrications. When you resist comparing yourself to Hollywood idols and other false representations of sexual appeal, you can shift your attention, become more comfortable in your own skin, and confident in your unique sex appeal and attractiveness.

84. Live by Your Own Script, Dance to Your Own Drummer, and Sing Your Own Song.

You are a Great Lover because you rely on yourself to determine what is Great Sex for you and your lover. We are all bombarded by the media's version of Great Sex: two twenty-year-olds slithering around in bodies that have been touched up, beefed up, or synthetically slimmed down. Not only do these images reek of fake sex, they also create an illusion of what Great Sex is supposed to be like. Great Sex is what works for you—and you are the best, and only—two people who can determine this quality. It's about your satisfaction, your pleasure.

85. Romancing the Stone.

This may sound like a tired bit of advice, and I do apologize for sounding the least bit tiresome, however, this tip is so important that I would be remiss if I did not remind all of you of its absolute sovereignty in the hierarchy of sexual advice. Let me sum it up quite bluntly: If you allow romance to die in your relationship, the sexual soul of your relationship will die with it. The soul is the center of your relationship, and it's either light, in which case it is alive with energy; or it's heavy, like a stone, and will fall to the bottom in despair. Need I say more? Do I need to give you advice on how to be romantic? I doubt it. Each couple has its own special way of being romantic with each other. Just keep it up. And remember that romancing is nine parts planning and preparation, and one part execution. The actions need not be grand—because it's the thought behind them that has the most impact. As the following examples illustrate, luscious, authentic romance is the catalyst for great sex.

- For Audrey's first visit to his family vacation home, Howard printed a banner that read "Welcome to La Jolla, Audrey" and placed it in the front window. He repeats the tradition whenever she travels.

- Knowing Eric's love of cheesecake, Iris baked her mother's secret recipe and carried the sweet confection across the country, packed in dry ice. Eric loved the cake, but the fact that she had cooked for him made it even more special.

- Thalia traveled extensively doing international audits. Before she and Robert were married, Robert always managed to find out the hotel where Thalia was staying and make arrangements for a bouquet of her favorite flowers, Casablanca lilies, to be in the room upon her arrival. He continues to make this romantic gesture ten years into their marriage—even though he isn't there in person, when Thalia returns "home" to her room, he is present in his behavior.

- Having paid very close attention to her husband's car magazines, Deirdre bought her husband a Jaguar sedan for his fortieth birthday. When he arrived home that evening, the car was sitting in their driveway with a monstrous red bow tied around it. As her husband describes it, Deirdre pulled it all off in pure New York fashion: Since she doesn't drive, she put it on her credit card and had it delivered. That's what you call planning.

86. Never Embarrass Each Other.

No one but you and your partner know your soft spots better and nothing can drive an emotional wedge in faster than exposing that private area to the world. So whether you are in private or public, never embarrass your lover. You may think you are being *très très* witty in recounting an event or making a sarcastic observation, but you are merely being mean. So even if sarcasm is referred to as the sour cream of wit, remember the operative word there is "sour." To embarrass is to expose and discompose someone else, and surely that is the last thing you wish to do to your lover. Do you really think they will want to jump into bed with you after you've humiliated them earlier? I don't think so.

87. Maintain Your Dignity.

Maintaining and protecting your dignity as a lover is imperative for your emotional and mental health, but it is just as crucial to the health of your sexual relationship. Without it, quite frankly, your relationship will wither and die. We all need to have our sexual soul treated with respect as it is food for our relationship's soul. Paul was struck by this truth when, after finally deciding to leave a marriage in which his wife continually had affairs, was told by his father, "Good, it is time you got your dignity back." When he heard his father's words, he realized how he had lost sight of his self-respect during his marriage. How does this happen, you may wonder. In the case of Paul, he had been so afraid of the truth (that his wife had betrayed their bond), that he was willing to sacrifice his own self-respect. The good news is that we can always restore our sexual dignity by keeping in mind these synonyms for dignity: self-respect and noble behavior. And there is no greater noble behavior than demanding that you be treated sexually in the manner you prefer.

88. Diplomatic Corps in the Bedroom.

There is no place where your diplomacy and negotiating skills will serve you better than in the bedroom. The number-one diplomatic issue of the bedroom concerns the approaching of and requesting of sex—be the signal a kiss on the back of the neck, or a direct verbal request, such as "Tonight?" while the two of you are eating your meat loaf. Diplomacy becomes a factor in how you accept or pass on the sexual opportunity; simply put, if you are gentle and kind, you have a better chance at keeping the door to sensual satisfaction open. And when you keep your eye on the long-term objective of remaining happily and sexually open to each other, rather than on the short-term goal of "not tonight," you will be guided by what works best for you as a couple. If you are not able to genuinely be there physically, then take a tip from some couples who have a two-refusal limit before they meet in the middle and talk about why. The key here is to always try for a win-win attitude should you need to negotiate.

89. *Keep Talking.*

About life in general, the day-to-day minutiae, and your history. In this way, you keep the texture and tableau of your relationship alive. We are verbal beings. We rely on speech to communicate. Without this form of exchange, we cut ourselves off from one another. And this couldn't be more true (and more important) for relationships. It is all too easy for us to stop talking to each other once we get into a place of familiarity and routine, forgetting or assuming we know the details of each other's lives. Don't assume! Talk! Share! Be open and willing—don't wait to be asked. Be curious and interested. Give your lover feedback. And by all means, show him or her you care. Every day.

90. *Learn How to Compromise.*

When the going gets rough, Great Lovers utilize a powerful tool called compromise. Don't think of compromise as "giving up," which can make you feel that you've lost; rather think of compromise as a win-win situation. Each of you has "won" something from an argument when you strengthen rather than drain your relationship. What does compromise require? An ability to acknowledge, listen, and accept each other's point of view—even if you disagree. If you're comfortable with the Tip on healthy arguing (#93) and the dangers of insisting on being right (#35), then you're probably already familiar with the great power of compromise to mend and heal the fences we create—often needlessly—in our relationships. Jamie and Louis had a vacation conundrum. As Jamie explained it, "I don't ski and he doesn't do beaches. So we have had to find a compromise that works for both of us. We first faced this when we planned our honeymoon. We both knew that if both of us were not happy, then that meant less sex, and less sex was not an option. Now we 'blend' our vacations, and make sure that we both feel comfortable. Last year we went to Costa Rica, where they have beautiful beaches, but they also have beautiful rain forest terrain so Louis can go hiking."

91. Be Tastefully Jealous—Possess Your Lover Culturally and Socially.

There is something heartwarming about being able to stir intense emotions in your partner. Jealousy need not make sense on occasion, but when you are in love and your heart is vulnerable, it makes sense that you may act possessively of your lover in public or in private. Great Lovers know this is an honest and self-protective form of behavior that often states they possess their lover culturally and socially. When you use the possessive pronouns in conversation ("My wife" or "My partner"), you are not revealing the insecure, wild, green-eyed monster that gets all the rave reviews. Instead, you are showing the world and your lover that you care so much about your attachment that you need to assert this connection clearly and concretely. This is a style of jealousy that has a visceral honesty about boundaries and often takes the form of a gently possessive act, especially in public. The "Darling, would you like me to refresh your drink?" or the kiss behind the ear or a hand drifting around your waist as they walk by. They all make a public declaration that that person has permission to be in your personal space. The translation: "She's with me." Whether we like it or not, any lover with two neurons firing knows that people get jealous. Quite simply we are hardwired that way. So rather than buck what Mother Nature put into place, use it to your advantage.

92. Don't Push Your Lover's Buttons.

What makes a special relationship special are the nuances that we create together with our lover—the way we speak to each other, our pet names we have for each other, the secrets that we share that create the underlying texture for intimacy and growth. Indeed, we fall in love because when together, we understand each other so well, making each other come alive in ways both comfortable and unexpected. However, as many couples have admitted to me, the same characteristics that we love in our partner also tend to be the qualities that have the power to set us off. Albert and Charlotte capture the paradox of this tip perfectly: Madly in love since they were in their early twenties, they have always remained best friends as well as passionate lovers. But they also know how to push each other's buttons, bringing each other to anger as quickly as a match to a fire. All Albert has to do to make Charlotte angry is tease her about her thighs; all Charlotte has to do to make Albert angry is to remind him he had to take the bar exam twice before passing. They both admit that targeting these soft spots in each other is below the belt, even nasty, and clearly corrosive to their relationship. So instead of pushing each other's buttons, they now take a moment to figure out why they might feel angry—about work, about something else the other may have done, or some other personal issue having nothing to do with the size of thighs or passing the bar exam. Once they take the time to actually focus on the real reason they are feeling badly, then they catch themselves before making a critical remark that stings.

93. Arguing Is Not Always a Bad Thing.

Every relationship contains differences and anger. Every relationship has its fair share of differences. And from what I hear, some of the healthiest couples out there are those that let off steam every once in a while with a good row! So it's not the argument itself that can cause problems. Rather it's the attitude underneath the argument. What two people are going to agree all the time? Not even Bogie and Bacall, the Duke and Duchess of Windsor, or Antony and Cleopatra went without their fundamental differences in opinion, and no doubt some of these differences fanned the fires of sexual tension between these heatedly committed couples. It's only human nature that we have different, idiosyncratic views of the world and all of its attendant noise and nonsense. So it makes perfect sense that these differences can lead to disagreements, and even full-on arguments. Any relationship always contains two voices and no one voice is more important than the other. This mutuality is vital to the healthy give and take when two people are really communicating with each other. When this spirit of mutuality is disrupted and the balance shifts, so does that couple's receptivity to each other. So how do you navigate differences in opinion that threaten to raise a wall between you? You need to be able to keep the communication open so that you don't create emotional gridlock in which the two of you get carried away by your own anger. I mean good grief, imagine a life with no differences! You'd be robotic! And often the smallest things you don't talk about end up being the most troubling. So this means allowing for difference in opinion, acknowledging each other's point of view, and listening to each other's side. How does runaway anger impact your sex life? Let me put it to you this way: How are you going to snuggle up to your partner if the Berlin Wall is up between you? There is no shorter route to a sexual stonewall than when a couple stops speaking to each other—the inevitable end to an argument in which one or both of you resists acknowledging the other's viewpoint and accepting a difference in opinion. As Mark says, "Sometimes when I get angry, I want to stay angry. But I know that could make it really cold between the sheets." Instead, he and his wife Ilene remind each other to take a breath. "It started out as a kind of joke that a friend in California told us about—'Breathe, let breathing be your friend'—but it's something we got into the habit of doing, and it works," explains Ilene. "When we take a breath, we slow down and usually the fight loses steam and diffuses the situation—the problem is no longer that important. But we always crack up laughing when either one of says 'take a breath!'" Like so many things, shifting gears during an argument takes practice. It also requires that both partners be conscious and aware. Mark and Ilene take a breath. Other couples might use a signal—a peace sign, a hand in the air, an umpire's signal for a time-out—you decide. What's important is that you as a couple create an easily recognizable way to signal to each of you that it's better to walk away from the fight and let go of the harsh and angry words if you want to keep your relationship sizzling. Differences are a fact of life and the clearing result of anger can be a good, cathartic energy in a healthy relationship.

94. Fight Fair (or Learn How To).

It's no wonder that most of have no idea how to fight fair: we first learned how to impact our world and express our wants and needs at about age two, when we learned the word, "No!" As toddlers, when things did not go our way, our emotional and visceral reaction would cause us to blurt out our displeasure in an often impulsive, unrestricted way. As we develop, adding to our reasoning and language abilities, we may attain a bit more skill at expressing ourselves, but, for many of us, no greater skill in saying what we don't like or what upsets us. So it is not a surprise that here we are at thirty, forty, or fifty years old reacting like toddlers to something our partner says to us. We might as well beat the floor with our fists and cry! Instantly, we are flooded by our feelings. We might be thinking, *Why am I acting like a child?*, but we blurt out, "I don't want to go to _____", "Where is mine?", "Where are you going?", "What do you mean?" Rest assured, you are not alone on this one. To give you a graduate-level class in expressing yourself under stress, I have included an incredible resource list for "Fair Fighting" from Dr. Jackie Jaye-Brandt, an outstanding Los Angeles–based relationship therapist:

1. **Active listening.** Take in what each partner has to say. Don't plan what you're going to say. No reaction.

2. **Turn criticisms into requests.** Look forward to resolving the problem with discussion and compromise.

3. **Eliminate demands.** Always consider compromise. Remember, your partner's view of reality is just as real as yours, even though you might disagree.

4. **One issue at a time.** Be specific—it takes concentration to actively listen.

5. **One person's issues at a time.** If possible, save counterissues for another time to avoid diluting them.

6. **Present issues only.** Don't dredge up stuff from the past.

7. **No make wrongs!** Don't blame the other person and need to make him or her wrong.

8. **Resolution-oriented.** Look for solutions and opportunities, not problems.

9. **No scorekeeping.** Don't refer back to past fights and their resolutions or compromises.

10. **Take responsibility.** Assume responsibility for both your upset and a resolution to the problem.

11. **No sarcasm.** It's dirty fighting.

12. **No labels.** Labels are judgments that take the attention off of the here and now.

13. **Eliminate story.** Get to the bottom line.

14. Commitment. Be in touch with your commitment to your partner and the relationship.

15. No yelling or raised voices. They're counterproductive.

16. No assumptions. Never assume you know how your partner feels. Never assume you can predict how your partner will react.

95. Are You Clean Enough?

It's important to be hygienically aware. In many countries, Americans are viewed as being a bit obsessed about cleanliness. However, I will share that women in ten years of seminars reported again and again that cleanliness is next to godliness. How clean you need to be for each other is a joint decision and personal preference, so it's up to you to talk about your mutual comfort level with "clean." And if you and your partner differ on this score, one way to set the gold standard is to have it be about your finicky nature, not your feeling that your partner is a slob. Otherwise, you or your lover may feel a tinge of reluctance in getting close. The bottom line is that you both want to feel comfortable preparing for sex, wanting to be ready for sex, and feeling no obstructions to sexual exploration. Any tinge of reluctance has the ability to short circuit a huge sexual power line. Why chance it? If bad breath is an issue, have a mint and then offer your partner one. Or when you're brushing your teeth, prepare his or her toothbrush and hand it to him or her—a twofold loving gesture. You might also share how much you love his or her fresh minty breath on a certain area of your anatomy. You can also take a date-night shower, take care of unruly hairs (nose, ears, bikini line), brush and floss your teeth, and otherwise stay mutually presentable. And gentlemen, always remember to shave below your lower lip!

96. *Ask and You Shall Receive.*

How you ask for something is often more important than what you have asked for. Confused about how to ask? Find a trusted member of your lover's sex and ask him or her the best way to say something. That way you get the insight into how ears governed by that other hormone are likely to hear or interpret what you have just said. Emily wanted to have Greg do her with her vibrator because it is one of the most pleasurable ways for her to orgasm—but she was scared to ask him. She sought out her good friend Matthew, who gave her some inside scoop on some men's fears that a vibrator will replace them. Armed with this insight, Emily was then able to bring up her request to Greg so he wouldn't feel threatened. They've been happily vibrating ever since.

97. *Be Patient in Creating Your Relationship Even Though Being Patient May Not Be Your Strongest Virtue.*

Know that a relationship doesn't happen overnight. If you are in the relationship that you believe, hope, and pray to be the One, then know this: Take your time. Don't try and rush things. Ladies especially, put the calendars away. Resist putting pressure on yourself or your lover to say things or do things. Don't make the mistake I have seen so many couples make and marry because it is the "right time," but not the right person. Commitment and all its relevant symbols will come when the relationship is mature and strong enough.

98. *Great Lover Moment: Take Your Time.*

David and Helene, a couple who have truly one of the most romantic, passionate relationships I know of, shared a very interesting point about how we tend to rush into sex in the early stages of a relationship. During their first double date, Helene was deeply touched when David said to the other couple, "The thing that really got me about Helene was when she said to me, 'I need to tell you one thing: I am not interested in having sex with you.' That made such an impression—it had the double effect of taking off a huge amount of pressure and, of course, only made me want to sleep with her more." And Helene breathed an enormous sigh of satisfaction that came from following her instincts and not pressing the sex early on in the relationship.

99. Don't Be Susceptible to Instant Gratification.

This tip is related to the one above in that it speaks to the need to be patient in your relationship and toward yourself and your lover. In our society we are programmed for instant results, so it is often hard to resist the siren's call to fulfill all of our wants and desires. This is especially true when it comes to relationships and sex. Yes, we all long for the intense tangibility that sex brings to a new relationship. We think that once that "bridge is crossed," the deal will be sealed. But take a moment. Think twice. Be patient. Sex is wonderfully satisfying—only if the two people involved are in the same place of desire and expectation. And knowing that you and your new partner are in that same place takes time. So don't rush it. Aaron and Marcela echo this sentiment. They waited four months before they consummated their relationship. As they are adults in their mid-forties, they were more than well aware of what they were missing physically, but it wasn't until they both felt emotionally ready that they proceeded with their sexual relationship. When you both are ready to truly enjoy all that a sexual relationship has to offer you—emotionally, physically, and, yes, even spiritually—the gratification you encounter will be nothing short of stupendous.

100. Money Is the Third Dynamic of a Relationship.

Money is a live being in most relationships and can have hugely positive or negative effects on your sex life. For many couples, money issues can have a slippery and all-pervasive nature. Instead of merely concentrating on how the money is spent, address how you feel about money—in general and in particular—all of the time. And believe you me, it sometimes takes years for someone's true feelings to surface about how they want to handle money in the relationship. It wasn't until after their eighteenth anniversary a woman shared with me that she would rather divorce her husband than have a discussion with him about money. I had been listening to her frustration about their different approaches to money for all eighteen years of their marriage. When she finally made that statement, I said, "Whoa! Hold it. Have you told him this?" Her response: "I know exactly how he will respond. . . ." The bottom line: She finally told her husband her concerns and fears about their financial security and household finances and he had *no* clue she had been so anxiety ridden over this issue for so long. Big *no* clue. After thirty minutes, she finally brought it up, and together they slew a money demon she had never told him about.

101. Treat Your Relationship Like It Is a Living Thing.

We are attracted to one another because of qualities we each possess, and then we create a new entity called "we." This new entity needs to be attended to as a unique, living thing. We need to feed it, pay attention to it, and bandage its hurts. This is another tip that may sound as if you've heard such advice before. But give me a moment here: Do you think of your relationship as a living organism? One that needs strong roots to grow, space in which to move freely, nurturing to ensure its safety and peace of mind? Sandra and Barry acknowledged from the start that their relationship was its own entity. As Barry said, "We get invited to places all the time; but unless the outing or party is good for our relationship, then we pass. Before we got married, we made a lot of unilateral decisions about how we spend our time, but now we always make them together."

102. Support and Respect Each Other's Personal Endeavors.

There are two operative terms here that echo the comment "the sum of the whole is greater than the parts." Support of an endeavor is usually the first step in this equation and when the respect of that endeavor falls into place, the synergy between the two gives one's partner a noncritical space to pursue his or her dream or passion—whatever it may be. Now this is not to say you need to give someone carte blanche to do as they please without any regard to its impact on the relationship. Common sense plays an important role here, despite our free will to exercise our desires. So if you think what they are doing is horse patooties, tell them! That is as supportive and respectful to your relationship and your partner as high-fiving their other ventures. When support and respect for one's actions aren't present, there is an unspoken criticism that shuts off a lover's willingness to share and reach out to you as part of their world. Without such openness, you invariably shut off the physical sharing as well. The unspoken message is "They don't get me; they don't understand that part of me." This is a tricky arena, for often people will speak with "forked" tongues about support for a partner's work. Pay attention to the actions, not necessarily the words. As an example, a talk show host regularly told his girlfriend how proud he was of her business accomplishments and how he fully supported the emancipated woman she was (I know, using that term sets the stage for what's next). However, each day, after his early morning show ended, he called her office and became testy if she couldn't talk for thirty minutes in the middle of her work day. In other words, his support of her endeavors was conditional: he could support her as long as it didn't interfere with his access to her. I hear the same story from men who tell me the women in their lives complain they never get to see them. Unfortunately, that often drives a wedge between them.

103. Give Each Other Space.

Even if you absolutely adore your partner, most couples need their own space for a number of reasons—the least of which is a need for quiet time alone to recharge their personal batteries. So rather than worrying that they are losing interest, pulling away, or whatever you fear, take a lesson from a woman who learned the power of this in her own marriage. "One of the best things that happened for me and my type-A oil exec husband was his weekly art classes. He recharged and had something that was only for him, a truly rare experience. The best quality created by our time apart was the newness it brought to our sharing, in experiences, conversations, and people. The results showed up on our walls and in our bed."

104. Fight for Your Relationship in Times of Stress.

Great Lovers know that their relationship has an ongoing power dynamic, with ebbs and flows, and they choose to work together rather than seeing every crisis as a power struggle. So remember, in times of stress, work together, not apart. If you have ever fought hard to win something or to attain a specific goal, you already know the power of an unseen internal drive. It is this drive that enables Great Lovers to keep focused on maintaining their relationships in the face of upsets, job problems, financial disasters, stepchildren, in-laws, the law—whatever the stress may be.

One of the better examples I know of was a producer who, after five years of a happy marriage, inexplicably fell madly in love with another woman. The resulting events led him and his wife to separate for almost a year. And then they began the long road home, working very hard to heal the betrayal of trust, anger, and deep pain caused by the man's rupture of their marriage. Seven years later, the couple is deeply committed to each other and now have two children. When I asked him how he and his wife reinvented their marriage, he said, "Our marriage isn't perfect. It isn't for others, but it is for us and we have fought for it, fought really hard and because of *that*, what we now have is more dear, more precious, and more important for us than we ever thought it would be or could be." There is an expression that nothing introduces a man to himself better than adversity, and nowhere is that more true than in the context of a relationship. When things are all rosy, it is easy to coast. And goodness knows, we all need to coast from time to time. But life isn't always about being easy. Life for us humans involves challenges, and these challenges do impact our intimate relationships and affect the ways in which we love and connect. There is a bravery and a spirit in fighting for what you want and that spirit often wins the "war" for Great Lovers. As Marlo Thomas said, "You can't be brave if you've only had wonderful things happen to you." Great Lovers know the world won't always be great, but they have an indomitable spirit and courage and will fight for their hearts and their relationships.

105. *Listen to Your Little Voice.*

It's usually your heart telling you something important. Great Lovers are clear that they and only they know how they feel. That does not mean they live in a vacuum, just that they are guided by their own little voice and not by a public opinion poll of their relationship. Doug and Lauren met on frosh day of college and fell in love instantly. While dating in college, it seemed like they were charmed. But when they decided to get married right after graduation, suddenly there was a maelstrom within both their families. Why? Because Doug comes from a Catholic family and Lauren from a Jewish family. It seemed as if there was no problem when they were just dating. But marriage? No way. Instead of caving in to the pressure from both sides, the two of them listened to their hearts and kept believing in their relationship. The day of the wedding, Doug's brother even told him "You don't have to do this; I'll drive you to the airport." But marry the couple did. Doug and Lauren listened to their own inner voices about the power of how they felt about each other—because as Great Lovers, they knew that their brains will often short-circuit the importance of that message. Without being cavalier or inconsiderate of their families, twelve years and two children later, the strength of their relationship has been a role model for many of how true love can triumph.

106. Be a Great Toucher.

Our skin is the number-one conductor of sexual and emotional energy. Certainly our brains, hands, and other body parts are crucial when it comes to generating heat, but I am a great believer in the astonishing power of touch to cure ills, bring couples together, and continually ignite the flames of passion. Our skin is our largest sexual organ, so it only makes sense that our bodies enjoy and are meant to be touched, caressed, and kissed—all over. There is plenty of scientific data to support that a chemical response occurs when we touch, which is produced in our brains and bodies. But you don't need research to prove how important touch is between lovers. What is the effect on your emotional state when she nibbles on your earlobe (or other strategic parts) just the way you like, or when he rests his head in your lap on a rainy Sunday afternoon? Touch connects us in a deep, primal way. When you remember to really use this oh-so-powerful tactile sense, you will see this form of sensual communication resonate in every dimension of your relationship. By remembering to touch your lover in an active, meaningful way, you don't limit the magic of sensuality to just the time you are in the bedroom; you can carry that heightened sense of erotic connection throughout the rest of your day. By touching instead of talking, by massaging instead of tuning out, by kissing instead of burying yourself in the television or computer, you are continually building heat between you, and the payoffs are huge. One woman, whose lover lives across the country, has been so moved by the way he touches her in person that she can experience the same stimulation even when they are apart. "When we're together," she explained, "he is so magical with his hands; it's as if he knows just how to touch me, even when I don't myself know how I want to be touched." How does this magician work? When they walk side by side, he will place his hand firmly at the small of her back and gently guide her. When they sit side by side in a restaurant, he will kiss the back of her hand and then place it in his lap. He creates touch that *lingers* through the skin. Remember, gentlemen, you cannot touch a woman in a willy-nilly fashion; it's not the fact that you lay your hands on her that counts—it is how you lay your hands on her that makes an impact. I'm speaking about the energy behind your touch. Is your touch meant to be soothing, arousing, protective, apologetic, or erotic? In other words, what are you trying to convey through your touch? A touch can silently convey "I'm here for you," or "You look beautiful," or, of course, "I want you." Touching is not just a means to an obvious end; rather it's a measure of a lover's ability to speak different languages. A Great Lover can speak volumes with his or her hands, and with very little practice, you can learn to communicate with your lover in a language that goes way beyond words. For instance, if she needs comfort, perhaps try the standby favorite: a warm embrace. If you notice she looks particularly lovely that day and you want to convey your appreciation for her beauty, perhaps a sensual caress of her cheek. If your aim is to arouse, a light sweep of the side of her breast as you help her on with her coat can produce the effect you are hoping for. Remember that it is the continuity of touching your lover all the time that will make the difference.

And ladies, don't be afraid to show your man how you like to be touched. When I say this, I mean show him with your own hands or put your hand over his and show him. There are three reasons this tip works: First, most men enjoy watching women touch themselves; they get totally turned on. Second, your man will appreciate the advice. And third, you'll appreciate the results. So don't be shy: Show him where, how hard, how soft, how fast, or how slowly you like to be touched on your genitals or any other area for that matter. Here are just a few ways you can introduce touch into your relationship on a more consistent basis—before becoming sexual—that will only enhance the tactile eroticism of sex once you do get there:

- Sit beside each other when watching TV. It may sound mundane, but you would be amazed how different the experience can be when you are actually cuddled up on the couch, body to body with your partner rather than marooned on separate furniture islands.

- Give him or her a gentle squeeze on the shoulder when you walk by. As one client put it, "When my guy does that, I feel so loved!"

- If she has a stray eyelash on her cheek, gently reach over and brush it away with your finger.

- In the morning, as you go to work or in the evening as you're getting ready to leave, use a lint-brush roller to remove any stray cat or dog hair over his or her body . . . in the process, you may delay your departure!

- Do a Hug and Run—come up behind your lover and wrap your arms around him or her from behind as he or she dresses, is on the phone, or preparing something on the counter. The point here is to do it while your lover is involved in something else.

- As lovers do in India, on a very hot day, lift her hair and gently blow on the skin at the back of her neck.

- End your day connected like one professional couple I know, who, after six years of marriage, fall asleep while holding hands.

107. Turn Off the TV.

I doubt this tip needs much explaining. If the television is present in the bedroom, then you will feel more tempted to turn it on rather than yourselves. By removing the Magnavox from your room, you also remove the temptation to turn it on. You also increase your chances of entertaining each other. Television, especially when it's placed in the bedroom, where most sex is initiated, is a major interruption and distraction to sex. And Great Lovers know this. Do you want to share her with anybody, much less a talking box? If, however, the two of you want to watch television together, then do so in concert—holding hands, snuggled in bed together, naked—skin on skin. Make the watching not a distraction, but an intimate experience that you are sharing with each other. Soon, you may lose interest in the black box anyway and find far more enticing ways to spend an evening.

108. No Kids in the Bed!

Don't allow your children to sleep with you on a regular basis. This tip doesn't need much explaining, but it does require moral support, especially if you are new parents and all you want is a good night's sleep and somehow, somewhere, at some time, you brought your infant into your bed to quiet him or her. But now your adorable little one is almost two and your sex life has gone kaput! Yes, they are cuddly little bundles of joy, but, no, they are not meant to be your bedfellows. Your bed is reserved for the two of you: It's a significant part of your sanctuary, so you must treat it as such. If your child is between you, then you cannot be the lovers that you are supposed to be. It's quite simple.

109. *Home Is Where the Heart Is.*

Create a sensual atmosphere throughout your home. Take a tip from feng shui masters and know you need to balance and extend the sensual energy and heartbeat throughout the place you live. One outstanding way to enhance your love life is to look at how each room can contribute to creating the sensuality the two of you prefer. After all, each room is part of how you relate as a couple. Start with the bedroom. . . . Then perhaps use rich brocade curtains in the family room, or a sage green moire shower curtain in the bathroom, or place candles in the entryway. By doing something as simple as putting smooth wooden seats in the kitchen or a mirror in the foyer or hall as you walk in the door, you can add a new dimension—never mind create a stage for your own sex show. Whatever your choices may be, the important thing to remember is by creating a sensual atmosphere throughout your home, you have subliminally established the mindset of sensation. Should you wish to indulge in more sensations, the stage has already been set.

110. *Hug Each Other.*

As you learned above, any form of touching is a powerful physical force in your relationship. But a hug carries with it a unique power: when you hug your lover, you are going into his or her physical space—and this is a special right that you have as lovers. Here's an analogy: Only your children can call you Mom or Dad; it's a privilege that only they have. The same applies to hugs between lovers, and in my mind, a good hug has magical powers:

- after a good fight

- after a good cry

- after work

- after sex

- at the end of the day

- at the beginning of the day

- as you get out of bed

- as you get into bed

111. Create Emotional Safety.

This tip carries waves of wonder with it. When a man or woman is made to feel emotionally safe with his or her lover, the potential for intimacy, personal growth, and sensational sex increases exponentially. I cannot underestimate the primacy of this piece of advice. Just think of how important it is for a baby or child to feel safe: When a child feels secure in his attachment to his parents, he then feels confident and comfortable in separating, and growing into his full potential self. However, when his sense of safety is in question, and the child is left to feel insecure or afraid, then all of his actions, beliefs about himself, and the world around him are affected. The child becomes compromised. In terms of our sexual relationships with our partners, the same cause-and-effect holds true. If you as partners do not feel emotionally safe with each other, then you immediately compromise the integrity of your relationship, shorten its potential for growth, and seriously undermine its strengths. In order to make sure you are enabling this quality of safety, ask yourselves these questions:

- Do you trust your partner with confidences?

- Do you feel you can tell your partner anything?

- Is it your partner you turn to in times of stress or crisis?

- Is your partner familiar with your emotional issues or your baggage?

If you can answer these questions in the affirmative, then it stands to reason that you and your partner share a high degree of emotional safety. If not, then there may be some work to do in the trust area. I'm not a therapist, but I can see a fly in the ointment.

112. Gentlemen, Remember That Your Fingers and Hands Are a Wonderful Source of Pleasure for Your Lady.

As much as women enjoy penetration during intercourse, they absolutely love the play of your fingers—everywhere. As you will see in the Playbook and in the Classics sections, there are many hand maneuvers you can employ to keep your lady on the edge of her seat, so to speak. But for now, keep in mind only one thing: Never stop using your hands to delight her.

113. Turn Complaints into Requests.

Let's face it, no matter how much in love, how devoted we are, or how committed we feel, we all possess pet peeves about our significant others. It's a fact of life: No one (including our very selves) is perfect. We all possess foibles, attitudes—and although we are often loath to admit it—even some truly annoying habits. So in order to communicate effectively, keeping the bad feelings from seeping into your sexual relationship, follow another golden tidbit coming from Jackie Jaye-Brandt: learn how to turn complaints into requests. Without fail, all the women and men I spoke with attest to the power of this simple rule of behavior. As Mary Kate and Joe told me, "We had to figure out a way to ask that something be changed. Joe is a fast driver—I mean really fast, and it terrified and upset me. But I didn't know how to get him to slow down. I would resort to complaining. But it was like he didn't hear me—instead of slowing down, he seemed to speed up! I had to figure out a way to let him know how important this was to me."

As Mary Kate suggests, complaining is not a constructive way to make someone change a behavior or an annoying habit. It usually just exacerbates the issue because the person hearing the complaint is distracted by the demanding tone or whiny voice. If you want to be heard by your partner, and you want your partner to listen and agree to change something, you first need to present a request rather than a complaint. But in order to reinforce this strategy, you need to come to an agreement. Mary Kate and Joe created an agreement that worked for both of them: Whenever Joe seems to be driving too fast, or in a way that makes Mary Kate uncomfortable, she asks, "Can we remember our agreement?" Instead of complaining, she makes a request. Now he is much more able to hear what she's saying and respond without feeling defensive or irritated. When lovers turn into complainers, they push each other away. Life is busy and stressful enough, and it's too easy to drive a giant wedge between you. It's always better in the long run to take the time to ask. But learning how to request instead of complain takes energy, forethought, and control of impulse.

Consider the following chart:

COMPLAINTS	REQUESTS
"Why do I always have to clean up?"	"It would really mean a lot to me if you took out the garbage."
"Your hands are way too cold."	"It feels so much better when you warm your hands before touching me."
"You never initiate sex."	"I love it when you seduce me."
"I don't feel I matter to you."	"When you make me feel special, I feel so connected to you—all I want to do is jump on you."

"You're always hanging out with your friends—I never see you!"	"I love our times together—they're so important to me."
"I hate sex in the morning!"	"I feel like I have yucky mouth in the morning. But after a shower, now that's another matter."
"You're so mean to my mother!"	"Hon, would you mind being more patient with my mother—I know she can be a pain, but it would mean a lot."
"We never talk!"	"Let's try to talk to each other; it's so important to stay close."

Complaints put distance between you and your partner; requests bring you together. If you make a request, instead of a complaint, I bet you'd not only get your way, you will see how this skill is transferable to a lot of other areas of your life.

114. Create Important Moments and Make Memories.

Seasoned lovers have the knack for creating an ongoing history by paying attention to their important sexual moments and memories. These lovers need merely dip into their memory banks to fuel, refuel, and jumpstart their sex lives. And obviously, the more personal and subjective the better. So whether you simply return mentally to the first time she swallowed, used novelties, or he gave her a G spot orgasm, Great Lovers never overlook the treasure trove these moments can provide. For Erica, hitting the Rewind button happened while she was grocery shopping and saw sprigs of fresh mint—exactly like the one she took from his Derby Day mint julep in Lexington, just before refreshing him in the back of the Jockey Club with her newly minty mouth.

115. Make Your Lover Laugh.

Have you ever watched couples who have the gift of making each other laugh? It is a bit like being a social voyeur: There is something down-right magnetic about watching someone trigger their partner's unseen pleasure points. Without a doubt, laughter is one of the best aphrodisiacs. When someone can tap into your sense of humor, they unwittingly make you feel connected. This connecting tissue creates an energy that is all at once cathartic, healing, and especially bonding. They get you and you know that they will likely continue to get you. For the majority of men I have spoken with over the last decade, one of the sweeter sounds for them is hearing their ladies laugh, which is made all the sweeter when it was them who made her laugh. "You cannot imagine how it makes me feel. I love to hear her laugh." And as another Great Lover sagely observed, "When you can make your woman laugh, you are halfway to bed."

116. Friends and Family Matter.

Create a special group of people with whom you can share in the plea-sure and triumphs and joys of your relationship. Let's face facts here: We humans are social creatures and we need more than just one person in our lives—even if you consider your partner your one-and-only, your lover, and your best friend all rolled into one. It's just not possible for any one person to be all things to all people. Great Lovers know they also need an ongoing hammock of support to occasionally rest in, revel in, and share their relationship with, especially in the beginning phases of a relationship. By developing and nurturing a special group of people to whom you can turn, share with, and invite into your life and relationship, you empower your relationship with reciprocal ham-mocks of support. This is not about setting up a regular opinion poll and group of "yes men," who will parrot what they think you want to hear. Rather, this is a comforting group of people who have a clear vision of friendship and honestly want to be there for you. Invite your friends and family to acknowledge and share in the pleasures and success of your relationship. This tip is so simple yet it's so powerful. The one place we can get the most heartfelt support is our circle of family and close friends. It goes without saying that our families and friends want the best for us, but we often overlook them as positive support sources for our relationships. You know they want our little hearts to be happy, so turn to them for strength and support for your relationship.

117. Allow Your Partner to Take Credit for Stories, without Correction or Editing.

This tip is related to the "be nice" category of how to fashion Great Lover behavior. For most long-term couples there are the standard stories that get trotted out to highlight their lives or amuse the crowds; all of us have a thespian in us. It's likely that over a period of time, each couple's stories have been embellished upon, changed at the discretion of the teller, and sometimes credit for the story is often assumed— inaccurately. However, Great Lovers allow each other to make such changes or to assume such credit without making a fuss. Why bother correcting your partner? Do you really want to say, "I believe that was me who . . ."? What do you gain by publicly editing the story just told—slightly erroneously—by your lover? Aside from a fight in public, few habits make people more uncomfortable than a partner who constantly corrects or kills his or her partner's story. Now that is not to say the partner has free rein on content delivery; it just means Great Lovers save "discussion" of the accuracy factor until they are in private.

118. Spend Time Alone.

This means spending time with yourself only. Whether you enjoy reading, hiking, going to the movies, meditating, or simply hanging out at home twiddling your thumbs, alone time nourishes your soul and spirit. Face it, no matter how close we feel to those we love, as human beings someone's presence always affects us. When we are by ourselves in a physical space, we relax in a way that is deep and profound. Such inner relaxation settles us, restores us, and energizes us. It's often very difficult to find this private time—we all have many obligations—work, family, and keeping up with our household errands. However, you as a couple need to establish the premise that without the time to be good to your individual selves, you cannot be good to someone else. This way, you can alternate on taking care of the kids, for example, and when it's your turn for private time, you don't have to worry about hurting your partner's feelings—he or she will understand and accept how important this is to you and your relationship.

119. Spend Time Alone, Together.

Just as an individual you benefit from alone time, so do you as a couple. Doing things as a family or with friends can be wonderful—stimulating, enjoyable, fun—but spending time alone, as a couple—allows the same degree of healing that alone time does for the individual. And I don't mean you and your lover have to be *doing* anything of import or substance. One couple, Ted and Alice, use their time together to sit on the sofa across from each other with their feet touching, reading their favorites. Another couple, Liz and Michael, love to be outdoors, in their backyard: Liz enjoys feeding the birds and Michael enjoys puttering in the garden. So the next time you get a free weekend, without kids or without work to do, slow down and think of how you can completely relax with your lover.

120. Dine Together Often.

Just as you put aside time in your busy lives to spend time alone as a couple, create opportunities to eat together. There is something inherently nourishing and enriching when two people break bread together. Seated across from each other, or nestled side by side as they do in France, sharing a meal as lovers, immediately connects you with all your primal urges, sex being the operative one in this case. Think of it this way: Typically people don't have sex with someone they wouldn't eat with. This sex-food connection whets two appetites at the same time.

121. Is Your Lover One of Your Top Priorities?

A relationship will not last unless both of you make your relationship one of your top priorities. The lovers who show their partners that their connection is important, naturally make more time for their relationships—whether that is romantic evenings for just the two of you, getaways or vacations that give you the space to really relax into each other, or lazy mornings in bed where back-scratching leads to full-body contact. When you follow this rule, you will create a trickle-down effect throughout your relationship: When you and your partner keep your sexual energy stimulated, you will also have more energy, enthusiasm, and focus for all the other priorities in your life.

122. Reinvent Dinner.

Have you ever planned a dinner in the tub, in a grassy meadow, by a pond or lake, at the beach, or on your own bed? Don't use utensils. Think of different ways you can present food. Here's an idea that is a little over the top: a Japanese restaurant in Manchester, England, began serving food on women's bodies. Just picture udon noodles over her breasts and sushi near the pelvic regions. The serving waitresses claimed it was part of a cultural experience. So next time you sit down to eat a meal, don't restrict yourselves to plates on a table! Here are some suggestions:

- use satin sheets to cover the table

- eat only when you are fed

- eat naked or in other revealing attire

- go au naturel and eat without utensils

- follow the Manchester model and serve food on yourself

123. Plan Trips.

An essential ingredient in this tip is the idea of planning. Taking the time to do the research, making the arrangements, and ensuring that the idea of getting away actually happens is what matters most—after all, planning and anticipation go hand in hand, so each plan you make creates more anticipation of potential sex on the balcony of the hotel, in the empty gondola, or on a beautiful overlook spot in the mountains. The other essential ingredient never to be overlooked is what a vacation, whether it be two days or ten, does for you as a couple. When you travel, you are more able to leave your everyday cares and responsibilities behind—just temporarily. Whether a weekend of skiing, a drive to a bed and breakfast, a full-blown Caribbean resort getaway, or an outdoor adventure trip, it will bring the two of you closer, create a new environment for the two of you to explore together, and will create memories. And as one man I know says, "Hotel sex is the best!" so even if you can't plan a long trip, just book a hotel room downtown and spend the night. The change of scene will add quite a spark to your week, and to your sex life.

124. Plan Outings.

What's the difference between an outing and a trip? An outing is a day event—a small trip that you and your lover can do in an afternoon. But the idea again is the pleasure derived from getting away from home and enjoying an adventure together. An outing could be a trip to the dog park, shopping for appliances, a visit to a nearby museum, or, if you're with the kids, a group BBQ with other families. An outing could entail anything—even a trip to the mall—that allows you and your lover some sense of leaving your cares behind for a while. Such departures have a rejuvenating effect and help balance the busyness of our daily lives, during which it's so easy to feel overwhelmed and distracted by our responsibilities.

125. Plan Sex!

You may think I needn't mention this tip. You may think planning sex is either too obvious or too unnecessary. It's neither. You may not be aware of this, but it's true nonetheless: all of us tend to plan sex when we are first dating or getting together. Why? Because we want to make sure it happens. And even when a couple has been together a long time, involved in a committed relationship, you still need to plan sex. Why? To make sure it happens. The premise of this tip came from an interview I was doing with *Men's Health* magazine. The topic was "how do we get back to the hot, spontaneous sex we used to have." I asked the interviewer what he meant by spontaneous sex, and he said, sex that happens on "date nights, honeymoons, vacation, or during college." My response was simple: "You plan it." And he said, "No, come on. There has to be more." I lifted my brow and said, "What was it about the types of sex you just described that was not planned? In organizing these 'events' you planned and expected Great Sex to happen." The key when planning for sex: Do your mental homework. If you organize and plan for sex to happen, it will more than likely happen.

126. Take Care of Your Body.

This tip is different from the one about keeping clean. This tip is really about preventive medicine: The better you are at taking care of your body, the stronger your body will be, the more sexually stimulated you can become, the more you can resist the effects of aging, and the more energy you will have. I won't list here all the ways you can take care of your health, but I will list a quick reminder of things to pay attention to:

- Diet—eat a well-balanced diet and make sure you include a lot of fruits and veggies, fiber, whole grains, and what I call clean protein. Be wary of processed foods and fatty meats.

- Exercise—how often you exercise is up to you. But try to do something regularly. The more often you exercise, the healthier you are. So be creative and find a form of exercise that suits you and that you enjoy doing. Even walking fifteen minutes a day will increase your lean body mass and decrease the amount of fat. It also makes you more fit and energized for sex.

- Meditation and yoga—relaxing the mind strengthens your ability to hold off illness. Meditation and yoga are known to strengthen your ability to relax, as well as boost your immune system. As a golfer, I can attest to yoga improving my drives and enhancing my flexibility. If activities such as yoga or meditation are too foreign to you, try some other stress-reduction technique.

- Adequate sleep—a general rule of thumb is eight hours of sleep. But ensuring that you sleep long enough for your body to refresh itself is sometimes hard to do. Turn off that TV, avoid caffeine after 3 P.M., and make your bedroom conducive to sleep.

- Moderate adult pleasures (i.e., alcohol, etc.)—a glass of wine or a mug of beer is certainly a wonderful antidote to a hectic day, week, or life. But consuming too much alcohol acts as a depressant, disrupts sleep, and can interfere with your life and relationship.

127. *Encourage Your Lover to Take Care of His or Her Body.*

Just as it is your responsibility to take care of yourself for the sake of those who love you, don't you also want your loved one to take care of himself or herself as well? You want them to stick around. Your relationship depends on both of you being healthy. End of story. Let your partner know that you want him or her to get and stay healthy. I don't mean badger your lover to go on a diet, nag him or her to join the local gym, or pester him or her to go to the doctor for a checkup. Instead, tell him (or her) that it means a lot to you that he takes care of himself. Encourage, support, and invite your lover to join you. As one woman informed her new beau, "I've waited a long time to find you, and your not taking care of yourself is simply not an option. You and this relationship are too important to me for you not to take care of yourself."

128. *Good Grooming.*

What does it mean when a man says, "She takes good care of herself"? He usually is referring to the care in which she takes to present herself well. But this tip applies as equally to men as to women. Great Lovers take the time to keep themselves neat and tidy:

- Regular haircuts are important for men and women.

- Well-maintained and clean clothes and shoes are important. Gentlemen, if you only knew how many women notice your shoes.

- Cleaning nose and ear hairs (especially for you hirsute men out there).

- Clean and tidy nails—you know where they will be! Whether you like to have your manicure done at a salon or you do it at home, make sure you keep your nails neat and tidy. Both sexes need to pay attention to their nails: If either of you sees nibbled, dirty, or chipped nails, you will not want to imagine those hands on your body.

- Clean teeth regularly—at home and by the dentist. When away from home, keep a travel dental kit with you—in your carry-on, your purse, car, or your desk drawer. These are available at the grocery store.

- Clean breath—bad breath is usually a result of natural bacteria in our mouths acting on the leftover food particles. Brush your tongue and roof of your mouth, as they harbor lots of food residue. Mother was right: you need to brush after every meal. If you are eating something spicy, try to munch on the parsley decoration; parsley's natural chlorophyll acts like a breath freshener. Where do you think Clorets got their name?

- Ladies, if you shave your pubic hair, be sure you are freshly shaved, as the stubble can cause abrasions on his shaft—similar to the way a man's stubble feels rough against your skin. In this case, waxing pubic hair tends to be better as the hair that grows back is finer and softer.

- When cleaning a woman's genitals, it's best to use water and a very mild soap, as anything close to harsh can irritate and initiate a yeast infection.

- Keep your genitals clean. The sweat glands in our groins are similar to our auxilla (armpits) and secrete a thicker, more viscous sweat that reacts with the natural bacteria on our skin to create "our natural scent." However, this natural scent can quickly turn into body odor if the area is not kept clean. Use the Rule of Mouth for maintaining the hygiene of your genitals: If you wouldn't go there, why should someone else?

- Ladies, most men want to smell the clean, natural you—not some concoction pretending to be spring flowers. This goes for overly scented shampoo, as well.

129. Take Care of Your Emotional and Mental Health.

Let's face it, we all have issues, we all come from dysfunctional families, we all have had our share of disappointment, hurts, and growing pains. But it's our responsibility to take responsibility for whatever emotional scars we may have accrued, and rather than attempt to resolve them (some are unresolvable), learn to see how they impact our lives. When we can see our issues with clarity, they tend to become more manageable and acceptable. And when this happens, the problems also tend to diminish. Here are some suggestions for staying clear emotionally:

- keep a journal

- investigate personal growth books and seminars

- practice self-reflection through meditation

- have a solid friend whom you can use as a sounding board

- if you feel overwhelmed by certain issues, you may want to consult a professional

Our emotions are the gateways to our bodies, so if we are not feeling ourselves, or feel emotionally "off," chances are we will feel sexually "off" as well. So be aware of the tight connection between your emotional health and your sexual health, and keep in touch with your feelings.

130. Remember to Speak Compliments Out Loud.

Are you aware that we have a natural tendency to keep our most complimentary and poignant thoughts about our lovers to ourselves? For a myriad of reasons, we seem to hold on to these wonderful pats on the back instead of sharing them with our lovers. Great Lovers do not hold back their best accolades and acknowledgments to their partners. My twin sister, Dede, related an epiphany she experienced in her own marriage when, as she and her husband were leaving a dinner party, Craig commented about a friend, "Carol is so great—she has spunk. She always says what is on her mind." My sister asked, "Why do you think that is so special?" Craig responded, "Because she is so much like you." Dede's stunned "Huh?" response then prompted Craig to explain, "Carol has that same quality that I have always loved about you. But she's only the warm-up act in comparison." So the next time you think of how wonderful your lover is, tell your lover. Don't be silent. Speak your compliments out loud. Great Lovers know how they feel means nothing until they deliver the message out loud to the objects of their fancy.

131. Gentlemen, Always Do What You Say You Are Going to Do.

This may well be one of the most important tips in this book. The Great Lovers of the male persuasion know their words mean nothing if they are not backed up by their actions. Whether that action is a phone call or a personal appearance, a man must always follow through on what he said he is going to do. If you say you're going to be home "early," then don't show up at 8 P.M., after the kids are put to bed. If you promise to take the kids to the zoo on Saturday, then follow through— not only for the children's sake, but for your wife's sake, too as that might be her only alone time all week. For women, one of the more powerful lines in the sand is when a man does not do what he said he would do. When this occurs, she simply eliminates him—in round one—so to speak. Simply said, if you walk your talk, you get action; when you don't, you don't. As one man rather succinctly put it, "Men can't remember anything they said, and women can't forget anything a man said." So it's best to be guided by the truism: if you walk your talk, you get action; when you don't, you don't.

132. Seek Out the Solace of Physical Contact.

There is a reason why they have volunteers take preemie babies out of the isolation of incubators and hold them. We humans are meant to be in physical contact with one another, it keeps us healthy and grounded. So in the quest for sexual health, keep in physical contact with your partner. Now isn't that a nice tidbit of permission? Be it next to you on the sofa, walking arm in arm, or placing your hand on his thigh while driving. This is more about connecting than PDA (Public Displays of Affection). You do not wish people to tell you to "get a hotel room." However, you do want to learn how to enjoy the feel of your lover's body and maintain a grounding connection with your lover's body.

133. Ladies, Go into His Physical Space and Hug Your Man.

I realize this may sound so obvious, but many men have told me why it is such a powerful physical statement. First, from a cultural standpoint, women control the access to sex so they are used to having someone come into their physical space for intimacy, in other words, they are used to men making the first move or overture. However when you go into his space and hug him (and I am not talking about a safe, sweet, two-point shoulder hug; I am talking about a full-body breast-squishing hug), you are delivering a very powerful message to him as a man from you as a woman. And these are messages that as a woman you wouldn't necessarily be aware of, such as, I want your body, I enjoy the feel of your body, I feel safe in your space. Ladies, this is a classic way to tell a man you want them. Samantha related what her man told her when they first were together, "Please hug me, just hug me. I have dreamt about you holding me." That comment stayed with her and when she awoke their first morning together, he was on his side facing away from her. But rather than get up, she snuggled up behind him and curled her body behind his. His body sigh, while still asleep, told her this was a good thing. Initially she didn't understand until I explained how important it was for a man to have his woman come into his space, to come to his body.

So this secret is about stoking the presex fires by giving him the very physical message that you are open to sex and wanting him. So any chance you get, approach him, take him in your arms, and press your body into his. In this way, you are entering his private space—also very doable in public—and showing others that you desire him. Men love other people to bear witness to your attraction for him! In a more private realm, you are also communicating that you desire him and relish his masculinity. And remember, no two-point shoulder hugs need apply; this is full-body contact.

134. Cuddle First Thing in the Morning.

This is a simple and straightforward tip. Just as I suggest holding hands or kissing before going to sleep at night, cuddle or make some other warm, embracing contact first thing in the morning. Such a simple gesture gives your partner (and yourself) wonderful, warm reassurance that all is right with the world. In other words, you are showing him or her how much you care about them.

135. Don't Go Looking for Trouble.

Have you ever been around those people who always have some drama going on in their lives? Be guided by their misadventures. Instead of acting like a cop in the relationship and looking for what's wrong or why things shouldn't work out, adopt a different viewpoint and concentrate on what is working.

136. Buy Each Other Garments That Only the Two of You Will See.

I'm talking about undergarments—but if a sexy T-shirt or black leather belt is what whets your mutual appetite, then go for it. As always, it's what works for you that matters. The idea behind this tip is to learn how to make that "let's have sex later" connection with your lover. If he sees you wearing the scarlet scarf, he knows tonight he's going to get some. If she sees you wearing the black turtleneck sweater she gave you last Christmas, then she knows you want to do her under the tree or on the nearest sofa. If he spots the gray, lace bustier peeking out from under your blouse, he is going to start to get hot. These are all ways you and your lover pass secret messages of "I want you" back and forth as a form of foreplay.

137. Give Your Partner Downtime Upon Returning Home After Work.

This tip may sound mundane, and to a certain degree it is because it involves a simple daily ritual that has nothing to do with sex. But then it has everything to do with sex. When either of you walks through the door at the end of a long day, all you want to do is relax—before doing anything. No matter how much you might love your partner or your kids, no matter how interested you are in what happened at school or the office that day, you want time to unwind and make the transition into the evening. Am I putting words into your mouth? Remember those scenes from movies of the 1950s when the husband arrived home, and his dutiful wife met him at the door with a cocktail and his slippers in hand? Well, I'm not suggesting you go that far. And I know only too well that it might be both of you who arrive home after a long day of working off the premises. But there is something in that bygone scenario that we often miss today: relax, unwind, meet each other face-to-face, and simply connect. You don't need a glass of wine or a beer to do so (though either can come in handy at times), but you do need the intention to allow for that transition time. Don't you want to be present when you're home? Five minutes is all it takes. So between the two of you, work out a way that you both recognize signals the end of the work day and the beginning of your together time at home.

138. Don't Keep a Running List of Who Did What to Whom.

This tip is related to maintaining an attitude of forgiveness. When we focus on how our partners disappoint or anger us, we reinforce negative energy in the relationship. This negative energy has a way of taking on its own life, quickly invading every segment of the relationship. You might begin by thinking, "Oh for Pete's sake, he forgot to take the dry cleaning again!" and soon you're thinking, "He never does what he promises. He's so unreliable. I can't rely on him for anything. This relationship just isn't working." I'm not exaggerating here. One negative comment has the potential to spawn many, like an airborne virus out of control. However, when you maintain a spirit and attitude of forgiveness, voice whatever disappointing thoughts you might have, not letting anything fester, then you accomplish two things at once: 1) you air what's on your mind; and 2) you give your partner a chance to respond before anger and resentment set in.

139. Take Pleasure in the Little Things.

The joy of this tip comes from the many little things we can take pleasure in—daily. I call these little pleasure moments green lights for Great

Sex. It's equally important to take the time to notice and appreciate these moments. The little things in life come from moments when you experience pleasure in how the rose bushes he planted last year scent the yard or the pride you feel when other women stare at your man walking through the door in the restaurant. Or the ease you feel when you watch the hummingbirds zip around the feeder while you wind down from your day. Great Lovers know it is the continual accumulation of events and history, the little things that give a relationship content and context, feeding life and breath into it. The pleasure you experience from even the smallest events—by yourself or together—helps to create a web of history that gives your relationship strength and longevity.

The Great Lover Playbook of Tips and Techniques

Great Lovers are familiar with a certain amount of knowledge of what to do—whether they perform those techniques with their tongues, their attitudes, their hands, or their most private of parts. Since Great Lovers have a twofold focus of pleasuring their partners and themselves, they make certain they explore all the potential avenues that can give them this pleasure. In this section, you will learn the best-ever tips and techniques to wow your lover in bed. You're going to learn great tips for enhancing how you approach foreplay, as well as tips to keep in mind for oral, manual, and anal sex. I've even included a number of suggestions on how to deepen the spiritual side of sex for you and your partner. These tips came to me by way of my many clients and were tested by my dedicated research team. I know they 'work, but that doesn't mean they have to work for you. Try the ones that inspire or pique your interest, and remember, always keep an open mind. You might never know what secret fantasies your lover has been harboring, and what sexual storm you may unleash if you happen upon just the one.

140. *Ladies, Know What Turns Him On.*

Knowledge is power. And in the case of sexual turn-ons, a little knowledge goes a long way. Let me cut to the chase: if you know that he loves when you let it slip at dinner that you're wearing your pink, silk thong for him, what's holding you back? If you know he goes crazy when you tell him what you'd like to do to him later, why not tease him a bit? Knowing what turns your partner on is a fast, sure way to keep excitement in your sex life. I'm a big proponent for learning the sexual cues that work best to get a lover hot and bothered. These cues don't necessarily have to be visual—like clothes, or the lack of them. Some Great Lovers know that simply saying a line or two can make their lover head straight for the bedroom.

This kind of verbal cueing is all part of the subtle art of knowing what turns your partner on . . . and off. For Zoe and Richard, it's all about hair. Zoe has long, wild, red hair that she usually blow-dries straight in order to keep it tame. But Richard loves when she wears it all loose and curly—he gets completely turned on, even though Zoe thinks she looks like a mess. "I love seeing her hair all wild like that," Richard says. "I know that she prefers it straight, so whenever she leaves it natural, I know it's a signal to me that tonight is going to be a good one!" (Zoe smiled knowingly as Richard said this, completely aware of the Rapunzel-like power of her hair over her guy.)

141. *Great Lover Moment: "My Dear, I Would Really Like a Slice of Pie Tonight."*

Over the years, I've learned that Great Lovers are able to communicate their unspoken intimate requests in public. Though the "code-speak" each couple creates is very individual, it's always fun and it's always important to them as a couple. Timothy lets his lady know he wants to dine on her orally by stating what appears to be a request for pizza, "I really want a slice of pie tonight." Of course, the woman knows it's not pizza he's interested in. In turn, she will tell him how she has a vicious craving for a certain dessert. Her request lets him know she wants to do him orally and swallow.

142. Gentlemen, Know What Turns Her On.

I'm usually loath to make vast generalizations, but sometimes I feel they are necessary and helpful. In this case, gentlemen, I want you to know that turning your lady on has much more to do with getting her relaxed than any move you're going to make. So how do you relax her? Well, that is up to how your particular lover can unwind and get into the mental, emotional, and physical state to be open to sex. Does she like a hot bath? Lots of cuddling? A romantic dinner during which you pay close attention to her? If you don't immediately know the answer to this question, then you need to do some investigative research. Here's how:

Step One: Ask her. She may have the answer at her fingertips, or your fingertips, for that matter.

Step Two: Try three options and see how she responds:

- draw her a bubble bath

- create private time for her, corral the kids for half an hour

- light candles in the bedroom or the bathroom or the living room

- hand her a glass of wine or her beverage of choice

- offer to give her a massage

- combine any of the above

Step Three: If she does not respond to any of the options described above, then you need to do some more field research in which you make suggestions.

Once a woman is relaxed and interested—on all levels—then turning her on sexually is usually a matter of course. Here are a few more tips on how to move her from relaxed to aroused:

- linger in the pleasures of foreplay (see Tips #152–161 for more specifics)

- touch her everywhere but her genitals

- treat her to the sensations of your tongue

143. Gentlemen, Know What Turns Her Off.

Great Lovers also know that it's just as important to know what turns their partners off sexually. Why? Not to state the obvious, but to avoid turning them off, of course! Now I know that sounds like common sense—why would anyone knowingly try to turn off his or her partner? You may be surprised to discover that many men have told me that even though they know something (like nipple pinching) turns women off, they continue to do it. Perhaps they are not completely conscious (akin to being half asleep) that they are doing this, or they are programmed visually from other sources that this move works. However, gentlemen, if you want to be a Great Lover, and have the best sex of your life, there is no place for such indirect, unthinking practices. You need to find out what your lover dislikes and consciously avoid those things. Sabine said that her ex-boyfriend Sam used to have this annoying habit of wearing sweaters when they went out. Why was this annoying? Because Sabine had told him again and again how sexy he looked in button-down shirts. She found it very arousing to see his chest hair peeking out over the top of his button. Why would Sam have continued to wear something that had the effect of turning off his girl-friend? Who knows? But for Sabine, the message was clear: "He was being rather dense. He wouldn't connect the dots—if he wore a tailored shirt that made him look so handsome, I was surely going to be more in the mood for sex!" It's up to you to take care of your feelings (whatever their source) directly, and use your knowledge about your partner constructively, playfully, and in the spirit of making the relationship thrive and sizzle—not falter and fizz out.

One couple was able to come to a compromise. Jeff knew his girlfriend, Michelle, hated the way he smelled the day after a night of drinking scotch with his buddies. She refused to go near him and even made him sleep on the couch at times. Jeff didn't want to give up those evenings, but he also didn't want to turn Michelle off, so he did the next best thing—he switched to vodka, which is odorless. As Michelle remarked, "He may smell a bit medicinal, but it's a far cry from sour scotch." Bottom line: the more you know about what turns your partner on, the hotter your sex life will be. In this case, knowledge is an aphrodisiac.

144. Gentlemen, Get Connected.

What's the biggest turn-on for most women? Years and years of listening to women speak about what really turns them on has yielded a winning response: connectedness. So, gentlemen, the next time you really want to have sex, and really want to turn on your partner, then you need to focus on how to make her feel connected to you. Sometimes all it takes is that uplifted glance you give her. One couple shared with me that he touches his lips to the side of his hand to bid her a morning adieu at the door. Regardless of how frantic your day gets, a Great Lover always takes your call with a greeting of "Hello, Darling" in that special voice reserved just for your lover. Now, this is not a one-shot deal. And it does require that you already know your partner—emotionally, mentally, and physically. But assuming you've done your Great Lover homework already (and there are plenty of tips herewith that can serve as CliffsNotes!), you are ready to roll and keep on rolling.

145. Gentlemen, Love Her Body.

If you are already connected, you now need to tap into her next biggest turn-on: Show her that you love her body. How do you do so? Well, start verbally. Women are verbal creatures. They like to talk, they enjoy language. If a man tells a woman that he loves her body—either one of its parts or its wondrous whole—her libido is instantly piqued! Once you have her attention in a positive fashion, then begin to show her how you feel about her body. Let your hands and fingers caress every part of her, trying to retain eye contact as you roam. And if she hasn't already mounted you, likely she will soon.

146. Great Lover Moment: The Truth Is in the Photos.

I read an article years ago by a therapist about what is revealed in a photograph of a couple. If a couple is comfortable in each other's presence, it is captured in photos. You will see an ease in how their bodies touch and relate, like an unspoken confirmation of their physical connection. Looking at photos of couples—famous or not—in the tabloids becomes quite an interesting event. The proof of a couple's connection is always in the picture.

147. Gentlemen, Stay Connected During the Day.

This tip is about laying the groundwork for one of the main ways women get turned on sexually: by feeling connected to their lover. This connected feeling is not, however, like a faucet that you turn on and off when needed. Instead, it's about a continual attitude and behavior in which you let your lover feel your connection to her. Here are a few simple tips to keep her feeling connected throughout the day:

- call her at work or home and ask her to meet you in a nearby park for a midday walk

- start her day by making her a latte while she is in the shower

- send frequent and funny e-mails that only the two of you will understand and appreciate

- send her a stuffed animal or flowers, "just because"

- bring home her favorite take-out

The key here is communicating to her that you've been thinking about her and your relationship; the result will be her feeling more trusting of your connection now and more interested in sharing her body with you later.

148. Ladies, Know What Turns Him Off.

I am going to go out on a limb and say there are two things that men have shared with me that are invariably blanket turn-offs for them. 1) Women who let themselves go, who no longer care about what they look like and 2) Angry women. Just as there are women out there with idiosyncrasies, there are men with idiosyncrasies. My point is that there are far fewer things you can do that will completely turn off your man (women are much more picky) if you are approaching him in a spirit that lets him know you want him sexually, you need him sexually, and you are going to have him sexually.

149. What Are Your Three Hot Buttons?

On a regular basis, share with each other a list of the top three areas of your body you like having attended. Do you like to be stroked up and down your arms? Do you like to be gently nuzzled on the back of your neck? Do you like it when he or she uses his or her tongue on the inside of your legs? Tell him. Tell her. Tell each other. The mere telling gives you more access, and the remembered actions, when revisited, will have even more impact. Some couples even use Band-Aids to mark what areas they want attended. And keep this in mind: Our hot spots tend to change, like the weather. So keep asking and keep sharing.

150. Create Your Own Love-Life Response Sheet.

You movie fans may get this tip more quickly than others. Have you ever been to a movie and received a performance review sheet to fill out after you've seen the film, asking you your responses on certain aspects of the film? Here is the way you can put together your own love-life response sheet. Start by doing a five or ten minute exercise in which you and your partner—outside your bedroom—individually write down what turns you on and off sexually. Then share your responses—you may be completely surprised, amazed, and even amused. Tell each other the things your lover does that turn you on. Is it the way his or her skin still feels moist just out of the shower? Do you go wild when he uses the shower head on you? Or when she gently rubs your sore neck in the car on the way home? Are there specific techniques or types of foreplay you respond to? Again, the more the two of you know about the other, the more you can do for each other.

151. Show-and-Tell for Grown-Ups.

Share with your partner specific areas of his or her body that turn *you* on. This tip requires you to point directly to an area and make contact. What is it about *him* that turns you on: Is it the hair on his arms? The curl of his eyelashes? How his wrists look in French cuffs? Ladies, show him. Touch him. Let him know what turns you on. What is it about *her* that turns you on? Is it the dimples on the crest of her buttocks? The way the side of her face catches the sunlight? Is it the way she rests her head on her hand when she eats cereal in the morning? It's show-and-tell for grown-ups.

152. Linger in the Pleasures of Foreplay.

As you know, 90 percent of foreplay happens outside of the bedroom. You also probably know that the more comfortable couples become with each other, the more they tend to "cut to the chase" and get right down to having sex. But if you'll remember, when you first met, most of that passion that energized the two of you came from the long build-up *before* sex actually happened. We take our time in foreplay at the beginning of a relationship because we are not as sure about the outcome; so naturally, we work a little harder at making sure our partner is aroused before we take the plunge. The next nine tips are specific suggestions you can use to whet your lover's appetite for sex. These have passed the no-fail zone of my research team because they are a careful blend of strategy and sizzle. And remember, ladies and gentlemen, that the longer lovers linger in the pleasures of foreplay, the more luscious the results of the sexual encounter.

153. Window Dressing for Undressing—for Him

Ladies, this tip will have him undressing in the foyer: Leave a specific garment in a strategic place for your partner to find. You know what your man likes, so choose a piece from your closet or your favorite dresser drawer and plant it in a special place so that only he sees it. Be selective both in what you choose and where you place it. First, he needs to understand in one nanosecond what the garment means: You want to have sex with him soon. And secondly, choose a strategic location that is in his line of sight (preferably when he walks into the house, the bedroom, or even his closet), and not visible to any children who may be clamoring for his attention. As you know by now, should a piece of lingerie be your selection, some men like lace and frills; others like black, slinky, silky garments; others like lingerie that is made of leather—even rubber; and still others prefer plain, white, cotton panties.

154. Red Light, Green Light—for Her.

Gentlemen, women need to relax. Have you heard that before? You can't be reminded of this powerful fact enough: If a woman isn't relaxed enough, she's not going to be as open to being turned on and into sex. So knowing your lady as you do, give her a sign that does two things at once: 1) relaxes her and 2) tells her you want to have sex with her tonight. Here are some suggestions:

- Leave her a note on the refrigerator telling her to open the freezer. What will she find? Two martini glasses chilling—just enough to give her the signal.

- Once the kids are in bed, make a fire and put out two cups of hot tea or glasses of dessert wine. Choose whatever beverage you know will go straight to her head, and then her body.

- Choose her favorite sexual toy (her Rabbit Pearl Vibrator? Her Hitachi Magic Wand? Her Sleeves?) and put it under her pillow. When she goes to lie down, she'll know what is on your mind . . .

- Make an exception and turn on the TV in the bedroom: but to watch a sexy video together. Make sure it is something that will turn her on—not off. Again, this tip will work best if you know the kids are already asleep. There's a great resource list at the back of the book with sexy titles from which to choose.

155. The Sock Drawer—for Him.

I can remember to this day the scent of my father's top drawer—clean, fresh, and manly. It was his place. That didn't mean I wasn't interested in sneaking around in it, which I did with regularity. Most men have a particular fondness for their sock drawer, and as it is one of the few places they access every morning, this tip is a sure winner. As suggested by a number of ladies from the seminars, take advantage of this male sock-drawer bond and place a very suggestive note describing what you would like to do to him that evening or later that weekend. You already know what really rocks his world: So if you describe that act or scenario in ink on a small piece of paper that he finds as he dresses in the morning, do you think anything else will get his attention for the rest of the day? I doubt it. He'll never see his sock drawer the same way again.

156. A Call That Says a Thousand Words—for Her.

Gentlemen, call her and describe how you want to pleasure her later that evening. Whether or not she works in an office or at home, you are bound to arouse her when she hears: "I want you, I need you." Even if she is reviewing accounting charts, her body will register your need, and she will start her own slow burn. Here are a few samples that have worked for some of my research team:

- "Honey, where'd you put the ____? I'd love to decorate ____ with it tonight."

- "I can't get the image of you doing ___ out of my head and I'm fantasizing about you f___ me on the balcony."

- "I just want to bend you over the kitchen table."

But remember, she needs to already be relaxed. Such direct declarations may be met with a "F___ off!" if you don't adequately set the stage.

157. Anatomy Lesson—for Her

Gentlemen, give your favorite part of her anatomy a name, and then leave a message for that name on the machine at home or cell. When your lover hears a message, such as, "Hello, I am trying to get in touch with Gina," only she will know to what you are referring, and you will know for certain she got the "message."

158. Playing with the Mannequin—for Him or Her.

While the two of you are dressing in the morning, ask your lover to wear an item of clothing you want to remove later. Is it his cute boxers? Or is it her black, mesh bra? Her stockings and garter? Maybe the clothing item is more demure—such as the white T-shirt he wears under his dress shirt or the silk scarf he gave her for her birthday. This tip works at the subliminal level: All day long, your lover will be thinking about you disrobing him or her that night starting with that item.

159. Spectator Sports for Two.

Stand in the doorway, watch your partner undress, and let him or her know you are enjoying the view. How do you let your lover know she or he is turning you on? You have two simple choices:

- tell your lover: Say it with words

- show your lover: Say it with action by touching yourself

160. Dance Together.

Have you ever witnessed a couple dancing cheek to cheek, leg to leg, their movements syncopated and their eyes locked on each others'?

Dancing is fantastic foreplay. I am talking about dances such as the tango, the waltz, the rumba, or the fox trot—the dances that require some skill and a lot of heart. Such dances bring lovers together, often mimicking some of the give and take that happens during sex. If you and your partner don't know these dances, take some lessons, or just put on some sexy music and slow dance around the living room. The mixture of music, body contact, and latent desire create a great preview to sex.

161. Flirt at a Party and Leave Early.

Here's the scenario: You and your lover are at a friend's party. You split up, each going to one side of the room to mingle. Then you watch each other across the room as though you had just met. Linger in your eye contact. Let each other know you are thinking of the other—maybe give him or her a signal that only the two of you know. While you are talking with someone else, smile, and then let your gaze follow your lover's body—up and down. When you walk by each other, lightly touch his behind or her neck. Then when you're hot and ready, go up to your lover and whisper in his or her ear, "We need to leave, now." Your arrival home will no doubt be silent but deadly.

162. Learn How to Praise Specific Techniques.

If you love the way he kisses your neck; if you love the way she licks your scrotum while giving you oral sex, then make sure you communicate this praise. It can be as simple as a few words, and these words will go a long way to getting more of where that came from. Aaron found out the truth of this tip after he told his girlfriend, "I am powerless over that thing you do with your tongue." That's all she needed to hear: She now regularly sends him to the clouds while giving him oral sex.

163. *Learn How to Critique Specific Techniques without Being Hurtful.*

On the other hand, if you don't like the way your lover is doing something, then it's up to you to tell him or her. Does he scratch your back when you're on top of him? Is she too firm in her grip while she gives you oral sex? Does he push too hard during intercourse? These are all common enough complaints I hear in sex seminars, and they are quite easy to fix. But, again, it's up to you to tell your partner that X, Y, and Z don't work as well for you as A, B, or C. So when you do speak up, make sure you deliver the message gently and respectfully with options for what you would prefer. That way you get what you want and they get guidance. In other words, avoid criticizing the person and focus on how the person's actions make you feel. That way, your lover can hear what you're saying, change his or her behavior and not feel insulted.

164. *Fasting Leads to Sexual Feasting.*

Well, okay, you shouldn't take this piece of advice absolutely literally, but hear me out. As one gourmet chef related to me, "I used to prepare a seduction meal with a minimum of three courses and matching wines. But when we would arrive in the bedroom, we would feel too full to enjoy the lovemaking." Now what does this estimable chef propose? If you think you will be making love right after dining, eat only two appetizers and not a full entrée if you want to be on top of your sexual game.

165. *Garner Sexual Inspiration from Any Source.*

I don't care if it is the erect crispness of the celery crudites or the tawny texture of the hummus dip, Great Lovers learn how to get sexual inspiration from just about any source—from food to exercise machines. As one woman told me, "If I want to get my motor running, it doesn't take me long to get out of the vertical thinking of work mode and into the horizontal thinking of sex mode. And food tends to be an easy way to make this switch—I mean, have you ever walked by a bakery early in the morning and seen the smooth-coated doughnuts? All I can imagine is eating that off of my husband's body." A man told me he gets sexual inspiration for giving his girlfriend oral sex by watching the luscious lips of the female news commentator when he works out on the treadmill at 7 A.M. So here's my advice: Keep your eyes, ears, hands, nose, and mouth open to all stimuli that may become a source of inspiration for your next sexual encounter.

166. Maintain the Heat of Intimacy Regardless of How Many Miles Apart You May Be.

There is heat to be generated in the adage "Absence makes the heart grow fonder." And chances are, you can find plenty of mileage in verbal and written seduction as well. One long-distance lover stated, "We are apart two weeks a month so we do phone better than any 900 number." Given the vagaries of today's working world, two-career couples are often pulled apart by work commitments. There are two behaviors that Great Lovers who maintain heat while apart practice. 1) They find a way to always be in contact. "Even though we have a nine-hour time difference, we speak once or twice a day. Yes, it takes planning and organizing, but it is the one thing we both look forward to in our day." Which leads me to point 2) In those regular contact calls and e-mails, they share, talk, and *plan* more regularly: They share about their daily lives; they talk about their relationship; and they plan their next romantic and/or sexual encounter. They keep the juices going because they keep the juices flowing. Instead of getting on the phone and asking what each other had for lunch, you have to make the most of what little, precious time you have to make your connection as tangible and vital as possible. All of this active communication enlivens their intimacy and creates wonderful anticipation of being together. Great Lovers are always creating their own daily history together.

167. Make It a Point to Find Out How Your Lover Likes to Be Kissed.

I cannot begin to count the number of people who have told me they knew their lover was going to be great in bed by the way he or she kissed. I also can't begin to count the number of people not being kissed in the way they prefer. Unless you share what works for you, you can't expect your partner to know what works for you. No one is a sexual psychic, and we all need direction in the form of sound or physical assistance. Here are some tips:

- **Step A**—start by kissing your partner the way you love to be kissed. You can do this on any area of the body you prefer. Some lovers prefer soft and wet, some a firmer presentation.

- **Step B**—stop in midkiss, wherever that may be, and tell your lover how much you love kissing. You might say, for example, "I get so hard/wet whenever I am doing this," or simply "I just love the way this feels."

- **Step C**—then say, "Hey, will you show me what it feels like to be kissed by me?"

- **Step D**—follow desired kiss with reinforcement: "Oh, do more of that."

Repeat steps A–C as needed.

168. Never Stop Kissing.

Does this tip need any explaining? Kissing is the first and last way a couple connects. If you stop kissing, you stop connecting. You put up a huge wall between you and your lover. If you're still kissing passionately, then you probably won't understand why anyone would willingly stop kissing. This tip isn't for you. Or it isn't for you now, anyway. This tip is for all you lovers who get lazy and stop this passionate, simple way of communing with your lover. In some relationships, kissing is very important in the beginning, but as they settle into a routine or life together, the kissing stops and with it a lot of the passion. Why do they stop? Usually there is an unconscious connection between kissing and seduction, and some people, once comfortable in a relationship, become complacent and less motivated to seduce their partner. Great Lovers do not take kissing for granted, regardless of how long they have been together. They are aware of its potency, knowing that kissing is not only some of the best foreplay around, but also a hugely pleasurable act in its own right. Here's are a few simple tips to keep kissing:

- think of every sexual encounter as a seduction

- begin each seduction with a kiss

- make that kiss linger: move from loving, closed-mouthed kissing to more erotic, open-mouthed kissing

- experiment with different types of kissing: Eskimo (nose to nose), Lip-Sucking (gently take your lover's lower lip into your mouth and suck it—gently), Tongue-Sucking (gently suck on your lover's tongue), and of course, French or Soul Kissing (this kiss got its name because anything of a sexual and/or open nature was historically attributed to the French, but of course most nations partake)

- keep kissing during sex

- always kiss when leaving the bed, even if it is just for a minute

169. Ladies, Use His Body for Your Sexual Pleasure, Again and Again.

A man wants you to use him. I'm not talking about using and abusing him, but about using his body to create your own pleasure. You not only satisfy a deep well of his masculinity, but you also tap into how men become most excited and aroused: by seeing you excited and aroused. And what better way to accomplish both than by enjoying the body that turns *you* on! Countless men have shared that they literally tell their lovers, "This is for you, baby!", "I'm all yours!", "Do with me as you will!" Men have said that when their partners "use their bodies," "There is no bigger turn-on. I get hard just thinking about it." Translation: In the same way that men get turned on when you initiate, they will also get turned on when they see you more involved, engaged, and absorbed in sex. When men offer women their bodies, they are not offering just anything; they are offering the physical essence of their masculinity: their erections. Use his erection to pleasure yourself by taking the tip and rubbing it against your clitoris—or in whatever way gets you off. As one gentleman explained, "Before my girlfriend understood that I was asking her to do herself on me, she would always hold back. But then I made it clear that I wanted her to do it—not so I could get off—but so she could. It was like an entire door opened for us as a couple. It's no longer about taking turns pleasing each other; we are both pleasing each other at the same time. Our sex life went to a whole other level." As you begin to explore *his* body for *your* pleasure, try to let him know that his penis is a magical thing. In doing so, you are complimenting the heart and soul of his masculinity.

170. Set the Scene in Your Brain, and Then Create the Opportunity.

This guideline is mainly for those who feel intimacy should just happen, presenting itself out of a clear blue sky. Au contraire my dears, make your imagination your ally—be it about what you have done or want to do. Unleash your mind and let it become your stepping-stone for creating opportunities. And the beauty of being director, producer, and cast of your own sexual scenario is that it gives you phenomenal license. As Great Lovers, you no doubt already know that the majority of "opportunities" have a large, planned component to them. Here are some suggestions:

- Pack a picnic lunch and hide your favorite toys underneath the wine and cheese.

- Send the kids off to a relative or a neighbor's and transform your bedroom into a boudoir—red lightbulbs in the lamps, low music, candles, and, of course, the requisite velvet sashes with which to tie each other up.

- Have you ever imagined sex in a harness? There's a sexual enhancing product that will give you a truly weightless experience. This is a modified bungee-jumping harness, called Bungee Sex (Awarded "Best Invention of the Americas" at the 1999 INPEX—Invention New Product Exposition), made up of a bungee harness and a series of straps that you hang from a stud beam in the ceiling. Check out the resource section at the back of the book for further details.

171. Learn How to Transform a Quiet Evening in Front of the TV into One That Is Not So Quiet.

Step 1: The first step here is not sitting apart; instead, join each other on the same settee, chaise, or sofa.

Step 2: Play a DVD or video that sets the stage you want to attain. For example, try *Shakespeare in Love* and find the bed scene. Surprisingly enough, horror films are a hit because they heighten senses and make women leap onto their male companions. This woman-leaping-onto-men result makes me think it is only a little too obvious that horror films have to be a male-inspired film production.

Step 3: Cover yourselves with a throw or duvet to get warm. Then once you have created enough heat, remove an article of clothing to "get comfortable." Also, covers do what covers do best: cover so others can't see.

Step 4: Continue as you see fit. . . .

172. Initiate Sex.

Don't rely on your partner to get things started. Men want to be with women who initiate sex, just as women want to be with men who initiate. It takes two to tango. When you initiate sex, it shows him that sex with him is a priority in your relationship. It also shows him that you relish sex for sex's sake. Countless men have reported how turned on they become when their wives, girlfriends, or lovers make the first move. Why? Because men find this show of power sexy; it appeals to their innate desire to be taken care of, but with the added thrill of being *sexually* taken care of. They get totally turned on by the simple fact that you want them sexually.

173. Make Any Venue a Place for a Sexual Encounter.

Above all, don't restrict yourself to the bed or the bedroom. Almost every male client I have had at one time or another will reveal a treasured story from his past about a woman who completely surprised him with sex in an unexpected place. These stories become their favorite memories, and why? Because men love the combination of two things: a sense of adventure, and when their women are spontaneously overcome with erotic passion! One gentleman fondly recalled the time his wife gave him spur-of-the-moment oral sex while in the parking garage of the symphony while the other concert-goers traipsed by. Another told about a long-ago girlfriend who spread her legs open while sitting up on his kitchen counter, offering him a bite to eat. As one couple shared in a seminar, "When our kids are home and not yet asleep, we love doing it in the bathroom with the shower running. It adds an aura of danger and of getting caught—like we are still teenagers. It's so exciting!" So don't overlook countertops, stairwells, or the balcony of a hotel room. Or try the inside of a walk-in closet, but don't forget to cushion the floor with laundry—after all, you and your lover will be adding to the pile. Again, it's your attitude of exploration that is the key to pumping up the volume of your sexual encounters and making some steamy new memories of your own.

174. Ladies, Rather Than Rush to Clean Up after Sex, Whet Your Man's Primal Power and Leave Some of Him Inside of You.

This is another of those, if-men-hadn't-told-me-I-wouldn't-know secrets. There is something very primal about a man sharing his "seed," his most-male fluid with you, and for him to know it still resides in you touches and connects him to you as few things can. As one man said, "Every time I am with her, and I know this may not be politically correct, I love knowing that for the next day while she is out in the world, I am still there with her as she still has some of me inside her." And there is a pure physiological reason to maintain him inside of you and not break the spell of sexual connection: the bonding hormone that gets released during sex and orgasm—oxytocin. This would be Mother Nature's way of strengthening your relationship. Some women rush out of bed and into the bathroom right after sex—mostly because we live in a "neatnik" culture that has created a negative association with our bodily fluids. These fluids are the source of life—how could they be negative in any way? Furthermore, not only does such rushing away from your lover break the intimacy of the moment, putting a cold distance between you, you also unwittingly signal to your lover that you feel unclean. If you knew how many men in my seminars have reported how wonderful they feel when their lady lets that part of him nestle inside of her, you may think twice. As one man said, "It makes me feel that we are one." So unless you are using a condom, let him linger inside of you.

175. Gentlemen, Move the Target on Her Pleasure.

Women say there is tremendous seductive power in surprising your lady sexually. This is especially true as you try to enchant and arouse her. So, gentlemen, you must change your approach to targeting her sexual pleasure. As a golfer I know that you continually change clubs, adjust your grip and finesse your strokes; you need to do the same with sex. If you know that she loves oral sex, and you tend to head for this target, make her wait by spending time north of the border. This is not about teasing her mercilessly or not giving her what she wants; rather, it's about expanding the sphere of pleasure. Even though you know X, Y, and Z work, add A, B, and C to up the ante on the sexual repertoire.

- If she likes you to manually pleasure her, using your fingers, surprise her with the Shaft Sleeves to create a different stimulation—inside and outside of her.

- If she is expecting to make love in the male-superior position, ask her to sit on top of you so that you can look at her. Then ask her to lower her breasts onto you so you can gently suck on them.

- If you know she's game, surprise her in bed by tying her wrists with silk ribbons to the bedposts; then give her oral sex.

The idea behind this tip, gentlemen, is to get her attention by sexually surprising her.

176. Expand Your Sexual Library.

Go to your local bookstore (or shop on-line) and peruse the latest selection of sex books and then choose your favorites to purchase. Then,
when you are in the comfort of your own home, sit on opposite ends of
the sofa or across from each other on your bed, being sure to have at
least one body part in contact at all times, toe on toe, foot on leg, shoulder to shoulder. With two different colored highlighters in hand, highlight the intercourse positions, oral or manual techniques, or toys you
want to try, and have your partner do the same in a different color.
Then trade. Plan sexual encounters in which you each decide to try one
of your lover's preferred, highlighted positions, techniques, or toys.

177. Don't Worry about Making a Mess.

I mean, let's be serious, sex is moist, hot, wet, and messy. Sex is not supposed to be neat and tidy. Why do you think the line of products called
Bed Head even has a market? The inference is you have that "freshly-
f___d" look. Indeed, the messier and sweatier you and your lover become, often the better the sex. Both are a reflection of your being into
it. So just let go: of worrying how your thighs look (he's not looking—
I swear), of worrying about ruining the sheets (that is what laundry is
for), or worrying that you'll break something (go ahead and break
something . . . he'll love it!). This secret is about remembering to stay in
the moment—sex sizzles not because you look good, but because you
are able to get totally into what you are doing!

178. Develop Different Styles of Lovemaking.

Just as you have different appetites for different foods, so Great Lovers
have a range of different lovemaking styles. Imagine your most ideal

and favorite meal, now think about if you had to go out and eat that same meal three times a day, thirty days in a row. You would be weeping for something different by the end of that month. The same applies to our lovemaking, as even the best ideas are only best because they bring in a variety and spice that isn't always there. The following eleven tips explore the range of possible lovemaking styles.

179. Hide-and-Seek Sex.

Find one another in the dark, be it inside or outside you need to use all of your senses and especially your hands. Possible scenarios include what a golf pro and his bride did on their wedding night, played nude hide-and-seek on his golf course, it took three holes for him to find her . . . turn off all the lights in your house, undress in the same room, then one counts to thirty while the other hides. Music is helpful to mask sounds as you then proceed as desired, and no fair peeking at the motion detectors.

180. Silence Is Golden.

There is something so very hot about having to be totally quiet about sex, be it in unfamiliar surroundings, or when others are around. One woman related a ski week in Utah during which she and her boyfriend were sharing their bachelor timeshare with another couple. Knowing the other couple was mere feet away heightened their awareness of every touch, every slow move, every tight thrust, and made them very aware of their own sounds. The end result being they paid more audio attention to one another afterward to great benefit.

181. Blindfolded Sex.

Have you ever had sex blindfolded? This can work with either or both of you wearing blindfolds. A scarf, bandanna, or any piece of soft cloth will do. With one of you temporarily blinded, you will more than likely feel what your lover is doing to you that much more intensely.

182. The Pleasures of Comfort Sex.

In the same way that we all have comfort foods we turn to when we are in need of succor, most of us have a particular form of comfort sex. Great Lovers are great not because of their serendipitous moves, but because they know the value of deep, connecting sex that comes with our most comfortable routines. In my seminars, couples attest such comfort sex to be some of the most emotionally profound and fulfilling. As one woman explained, "Raymond and I have tried just about everything. But I can assure you there is nothing that keeps us closer than our standard sex. We know this horizontal dance, and like dancers who float around a dance floor, we know each other here better than anywhere."

183. Investigate Baby-Making Sex

Now even if pregnancy is not the immediate goal, you might find a hotter heat if you consider that each time you have sex, you have the possibility of creating a new life. For those of you who are interested in expanding your family, you know the fun of "practice makes perfect." I remember a study that showed one of the most erotic things for some women about making love with their partner was the possibility of being impregnated. Should you be in the practicing mode, all of these positions are ergonomically designed for the ultimate consummation while giving you position options. They are set for: maximum penetration by the man with the woman's pelvis at a tilt so that the sperm are deposited as deeply as possible into the vaginal vault and as closely as possible to the cervix for ease of entry into the uterus. This also ensures that the man's seminal fluid remains inside, while at the same time, the woman is in a comfortable position to remain in post-coital glow for at least five minutes afterward, thereby enhancing your chances of conception. **Position #1** has the most pronounced hip tilt, **position #2** has the man at a slight angle over her body so that during the extended after-glow connection, she doesn't feel squished. Note the pillow under her hips to maintain the pelvic tilt so the semen doesn't run out. And in **position #3** the deepness of penetration and her position both contribute to enhancing conception.

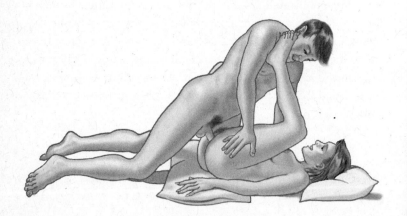

Ill. 1 *Position 1*

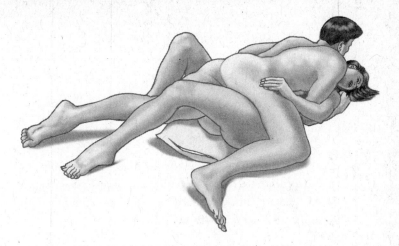

Ill. 2 *Position 2*

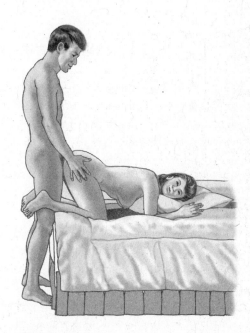

Ill. 3 *Position 3*

184. More Tips on Baby-Making Sex.

Here are some more tips to increase your baby-making chances:

- Linger over foreplay. The hotter you are, the more aroused the woman will become, which means that she can make her vagina more alkaline, and thereby more receptive to sperm.

- Her orgasm helps to move the sperm further into the cervix and deeper into the uterus for fertilization. This has to do with the involuntary muscle contractions that occur during a female orgasm or that follow shortly after.

- During post-coital glow, stay cuddled in a warm, body embrace. Such heat will just make the special potential of the moment simply last longer.

185. The Heat of "Pregnancy" Sex.

Many women have shared in my sexuality seminars that pregnancy sex was some of their best sex. Why? Because of the increased volume of blood (vasocongestion) in their pelvises due to the pregnancy. These women found it much easier to orgasm. Since orgasms are powered by blood and oxygen, the more, the merrier. As one woman stated, "I would give my eyeteeth to have the ease of pregnancy orgasms back." Some women also believe that because they were not at all worried about getting pregnant, they relaxed more deeply and therefore felt sexual sensations more deeply. In general, unless there are medical reasons not to engage in sexual relations, there is no reason not to. Once you get around the obstacle course of your belly and find comfortable positions for you and your partner, then you might be surprised to discover how deeply satisfying sex can be while pregnant—that is, of course, if you're not completely swooning with fatigue. **Illustrations 4–10** give you a range of possibilities to choose from throughout your pregnancy.

For the first trimester, the main factors that impact desire are being bone-weary tired and nausea, so the comfort styles of sex as shown in **Illustrations 4 and 5** may be your preference.

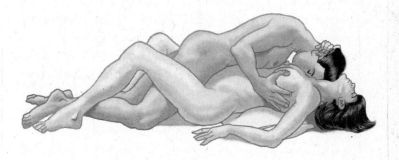

Ill. 4

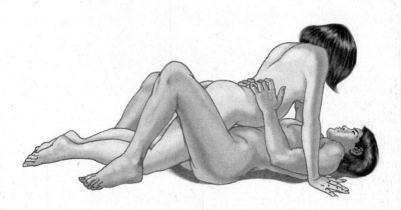

Ill. 5

As you enter your second trimester, you get your energy back and nausea abates and you have yet to have your growing tummy inhibit the majority of your moves. **Illustrations 6–8** present some mid-pregnancy options. In **illustration number 6,** the woman can control the depth of penetration and motion very easily using the strength of her legs. **Figures number 7 and 8** show the more relaxing-into-sensation positions. For all three of the mid-pregnancy positions, the woman or the man can manually stimulate the woman's clitoris if that is preferred. **Position number 8** works very well for those ladies who know one side of their vaginal vault is more sensitive than the other, and still allows the man an ability to experience firm, penetrative strokes for his pleasure. And as any woman knows, having your man in just the right place creating pleasure is a function of location, location, location.

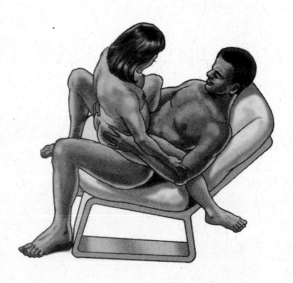

Ill. 6

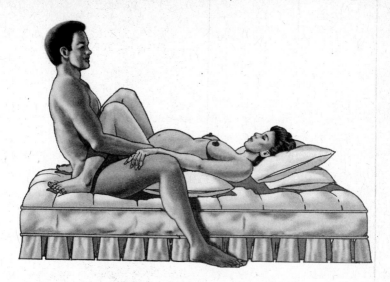

Ill. 7

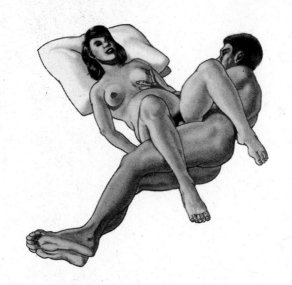

Ill. 8

When you enter your final (third) trimester, your options narrow as your tummy widens; yet this in no way takes away from your ability to enjoy great sex. **Illustration number 9** gives the woman the control factor while maintaining motion control when holding the headboard. Men who can't get enough of their pregnant wives' bodies have said they loved this position as they can watch all parts of her body move, especially her swollen breasts, knowing that because she is on top, she is doing everything for herself. **Illustration number 10** shows how a woman can relax into the sensation while supporting her tummy and still engage in a preferred position.

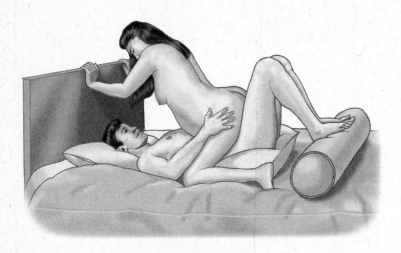

Ill. 9

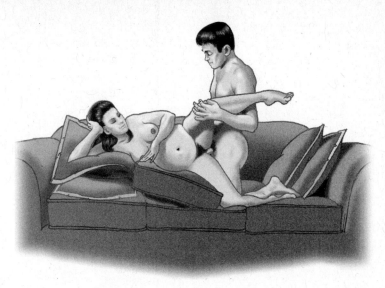

Ill. 10

186. Explore Middle-of-the-Night Sex.

Some couples who engage in this occasional style of sex claim its affirming value is the core nature of the act. For some it is a slow, gentle penetration from behind. Others move from spooning into a side-by-side penetration (see **illustration number 11**), with him creating their private style of stolen lovemaking, accessing her body as she balances on the edges of sleep. Of course, middle-of-the-night sex can be initiated by either the man or the woman. She may try waking the man up by sucking on him or moving on top of him, gently rocking back and forth to awaken his penis. Before attempting such sexual larceny, however, you may want to discuss the general concept with each other. If your partner absolutely abhors to be woken up in the middle of the night, chances are she or he is going deliver a blow, not a kiss, when spooned.

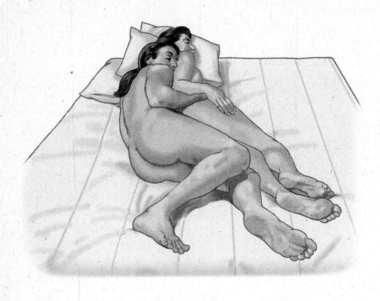

Ill. 11

187. Practice Children-in-the-House Sex.

One of the things parents become very good at is time management, which includes finding the time for sex. For some couples with children, they learn how to utilize 5–10 minute windows in very unique ways. Consider these options:

- manual sex in the car en route to get groceries

- sex with her seated on the countertop in the bathroom with the shower running

- a firm Do Not Disturb sign and lock on their bedroom door for midday retreats

The more important point about this tip is the attitude behind it: a flat-out refusal to let the fact that they are parents disrupt the fact that they are also lovers—and Great Ones at that.

188. Attempt First-Thing-in-the-Morning Sex.

Mother Nature actually rigged us to be best at sex in the morning because of a natural daily peak of hormones midmorning. If you are awkward with each other before brushing your teeth or showering, try a side-by-side position, with him or her behind. This position is warm and inviting, but not face-to-face. If the two of you get really aroused, you can always try intercourse doggie style. Just keep in mind that morning happens to be your natural sexual peak, so take advantage of this surge in hormones when you can.

189. Great Lover Moment: The Morning Erection.

Many men wake in the morning with an erection. Although this, too, is a part of the body's natural cycle, it does not necessarily result in a hormonal urge or desire to have sex. These erections are the body's way of maintaining the health of the penile vascular tissue. Just like the erections a man has during the night, the morning erections usually follow a period of REM sleep (Rapid Eye Movement), which occurs right before waking up. But as Bob and Claire learned, why waste a good thing? They love waking up to Bob's erection—regardless of its origin.

190. Relish Late-Afternoon Sex.

Some couples have shared that a late afternoon romp (usually on weekends) does wonders for their overall morale. Those I've spoken with say that there is a certain sexiness to this time of day, with the sun lower in the sky, evening not quite having arrived. This limbo allows for a certain suspension of cares and worries, a softness that brings them together in a sensual, soothing way.

191. Talk Dirty to Me.

Some men and women go wild when they are sexually explicit with each other. Tim told me a remarkable story. When he and his girlfriend were at a recent party, she whispered in his ear about what she wanted him to do to her that night. "I started walking into walls. Literally, I couldn't focus on anything but getting out the door." When I asked him what she said that got him so hot and bothered, Tim responded *almost* shyly, "She said, 'I want you to f___ me up the ass.'" Not a bit of a wonder that he was walking into walls! But know this, ladies: You are in charge of the level of explicitness. Many men like you to talk a bit dirty, but you need to feel comfortable doing so. See tip 311, Talk Dirty, for the fantasy scenario of this.

192. Sex in the Shower.

Sex in the shower is steamy, slithery, and slippery, and you have lots of props to make the slither even more slippery—shampoo, a gentle shower gel, even old-fashioned soap—but make sure it's mild. Here are a few suggestions: take a bath mitt or soft washcloth and lather your partner from the belly down. Ladies, he will love it when you gently massage his penis, using lots of lather around his testicles—remember to treat them like small, breakable eggs. Once you've begun to rinse him, and if there's room, kneel down and give him oral sex. Most men love the sensation of your mouth around his erection while the beads of water pulse down from above. Gentlemen, women love to be washed. Stand behind her and gently wash her breasts, torso, and her inner thighs with your hands or a bath mitt. The idea here is to roam her body without directly stimulating her genitals—they will be wet all on their own. Then ask her if she wants you to enter her from behind. One requirement: a bath mat so you can maintain your upright positions.

193. Sex in the Bath.

This tip requires a rather large bathtub and is best done with the woman sitting astride the man. Once the two of you have massaged and cleansed each other, all the while kissing madly to make the steam in the room even thicker, use some lubrication (Slippery Stuff gel is best under these wet conditions), and try for some slithery up and down action. Again, one requirement: a nonslip bath mat so you can keep your rhythm going without slipping below the water.

194. Sex in a Steam Room.

While most of us do not have a steam room in the privacy of our own homes, there is a special danger in trying to squeeze in a quickie at the health club—that is, of course, if you know how to be hygienic about it. An important point here is you won't be doing a lot of moving; this is a very controlled sexual encounter. Also, you know those small white towels clubs provide you with? Use them! Lay them down on any surface. If the steam room has multiple bench levels, then you might find intercourse interesting with one of you sitting and one of you standing.

The sexiness of this tip comes from all the sweat and slather the two of you make together!

195. Skinny-Dip.

This tip may not include sex per se; but it can surely lead to it! Where can you skinny-dip? Well, obviously, you have more choices during warm weather. But my point here is not to overlook the fun element of sex. Skinny-dipping with your lover can shed years off your mental age and do wonders for your chronological age. So next time you're near a free body of water, get naked and dive right in.

196. Have Sex Even When You're Not in the Mood.

You're two people, so it makes sense that there will be times when one of you may be in the mood for sex, and the other will not. Why have sex when you're not in the mood? Here are my chief reasons:

a. it will bring you and your lover closer together

b. once you begin, chances are you will be in the mood

c. the longer you have a "dry" spell, the longer you will not be lovers in the purest sense of the word

197. How to Get Your Lover Hot When He or She Is Not.

Here are some suggestions if you're in the mood, but your lover is not:

- If it's the woman who is not in the mood, you need to pay more attention to her. Attention is like sunshine to women: It brings them out of themselves, a secret every good hairdresser knows. Another way to help her is by removing those time-gobbling things that are getting in the way of her having time to get in the mood.

- If it's the man who is not in the mood, you need to get his mind off whatever it's on. Remember, men compartmentalize their lives. So if he is still thinking about work or the fact that the Jets lost again, then it's up to you to move his brain to you and sex. Try any of the foreplay techniques or begin slowly, manually stimulating him.

But the key for both of you is to try to let yourself go and surrender to the pleasure.

198. Explore Erotic Books.

Sex books are different from erotica. Classic erotica is more impression and narrative oriented, but it can get you just as hot as any how-to book—perhaps even more so. Some of my favorites are:

- *The Best American Erotica 2003*, Susie Bright
    This is Susie's tenth anniversary edition and once again she does what she does best: she has skillfully prepared and delivered a gourmet erotic buffet, the variety is such that all you need do is choose your pleasure.

- *Best Women's Erotica*, Marcy Sheiner
    The stories collected in this anthology are for the smart and curious reader; said to be "hot, sexy, literate, and thought-provoking," they deal with the "darker side of sex" says editor Sheiner.

- *Sweet Life*, Editor Violet Blue
    From naughty girls to dominant girls, from truly sensual massage to abductions as you please, from exhibitionism on the

subway to threesomes and phone sex with style, this is a we-did-it-you-can-too anthology of real couples playing out their fantasies.

Find a story you like and read it to each other in bed.

199. Read *the* Kama Sutra.

This is a centuries-old guide that claims to include every possible sexual tip, with exotic illustrations. You will find wild positions and varied and sun-dried secrets from the Eastern tradition. Use it as a source of information or as a titillating book for you and your lover to look at together.

200. Explore Erotic Movies.

Again, erotic films are very different from porn, especially your status-quo pornography that is aimed specifically at a male audience. Erotic films offer a more developed storyline and don't necessarily include footage of sex scenes. They are, in general, less explicit. But they do offer much more of a subtle, sophisticated experience that you and your partner might find very arousing indeed. A terrific video guide for female viewers—and great for first timers—is Violet Blue's new book, *The Ultimate Guide to Adult Videos: How to Watch Adult Videos and Make Your Sex Life Sizzle*. She highly recommends videos by female directors for first-time female viewers, especially Veronica Hart, Tina Tyler, and Candida Royalle. Their films are just on the other side of softcore, combining explicit sex with plot and complex relationships—no easy feat. But not all women want plot, some might just want to see hot sex, straight, with no chaser, and for those women she recommends John Leslie's Voyeur series and all-sex videos by female director Shane. The Voyeurs feature incredibly focused sex in twosomes and threesomes, with a gorgeous cast that is usually European. Shane is a college-girl type, and she gets together with her attractive guy and gal pals, and they go on trips (such as river rafting) and have sex in natural locations. There are lots of female orgasms in Shane's videos. None of these directors include any cheesy porn music in their videos.

Here are Violet's top picks:

(films with plot)

- *Tina Tyler's Going Down*

- *Love's Passion* (Hart)

- *Taken* (Hart)

- *White Lightning* (Hart)

- *Eyes of Desire 2* (Royalle)

- *One Size Fits All* (Royalle)

(films with all sex, no plot)

- John Leslie's Voyeur series numbers 7, 10, and 13

- Shane's World videos, number 19 and number 20

201. Feed Each Other.

Elsewhere I have mentioned how important it is for couples to dine together, how when they go through the ritual of eating, they are satisfying one of our most primal urges. The urge to eat is inherently connected to the urge for sex. This tip, then, is taking this connection to the next level: when you feed each other, you are getting that much closer to giving yourself to each other sexually. Order or make a platter of food—one or two plates that you share—and take turns feeding each other.

202. Eat Cake.

Or eat other aphrodisiacal foods of you choice. Here are some standard foods that we associate with erotic or aphrodisiac appeal: artichokes, oysters, and chocolate. But consider expanding your pantry with these foods, in these ways:

- Eat mangoes while naked in bed. They're juicy, so be prepared to lick each other clean.

- Treat her to a lollipop. You like the way she tastes, so why not place the lollipop inside of her mouth and then you lick the pop.

- Feed each other any finger food you desire, from Doritos laden with salsa to gold-dusted truffles.

- Spoon berries and cream into each other's mouth, using the spoon or your fingers to trace the cream around each other's bodies.

- Drizzle honey or chocolate or, my favorite, caramel all over each other and then lick it off.

- Pour brandy (or your liqueur of choice) in each other's belly buttons and suck it out.

203. Expand Your Sensuality.

You have five senses, so use them. When it comes to seducing your lover, you increase your pleasure when you incorporate all five senses— watch your lover, listen to his or her voice, touch him or her, smell him or her (all over), and taste all the different parts of him or her. The senses are avenues of sexual pleasure, and the more open and in use they are, the more aroused you can make each other. Think of the secret above: Sex is messy. How does it get messy? When you allow yourself (and your partner) to create and experience sensation using all of your senses. Touch with your fingers, taste with your tongue, listen to both of you hum or moan, inhale the scent of your sex, and watch it all happen, then you create a bursting bonfire of stimulation. After all, you can't have sensation without your senses. The next five tips show you ways to begin opening your sensuality together.

204. Stimulate Your Sense of Smell.

Any scent, fresh flowers, perfume, aromatherapy, coffee, pumpkin pie—whatever works for you—can impact your sensuality and therefore your sexual readiness and openness. So as you plan your sexual encounter, while you set the mood, make a point to incorporate your sense of smell. Spray yourself and the room with your favorite scent, light a fragrant candle, burn incense, or boil potpourri. By adding this element to the general sensual environment, you stimulate a deep reaction within both of you. Indeed, some men say that one of their biggest turn-ons are the natural scents of their lovers. If you want to explore aromatherapy, here are some scents that are known to be aphrodisiacal. They work on the brain to release endorphins—our feel-good chemicals:

- clary sage

- jasmine

- ylang ylang

- patchouli

- rose

205. Great Lover Moment: Take Your Love Away With You.

Kate, a recent seminar attendee whose lover travels a lot for work, told me a very touching story: When her boyfriend called her from Asia, after being gone for two weeks, he told her, "I have you here with me. I not only carry your picture, but the T-shirt you last slept in." What she didn't tell him that the T-shirt he had was her favorite and just happened to be from her high school reunion. What's at work in this tip? The T-shirt carries her smell, and breathing her in allows him to reconnect with her while they are apart, and for her it is like being able to fall asleep with him from afar.

206. Seeing Is Believing.

Given the incredible range of images available to us, it makes sense that our sight is one of the most evocative and proactive senses. A color may remind you of the red-hot thong she wears. The shape of a man's Italian jacket has you fantasizing about his broad shoulders over you during sex. Instead of concentrating on the usual images that get you hot, consider expanding your visual repertoire and explore areas you haven't yet. Why not peruse Shunga, ancient Japanese erotica, and look at what they thought was hot? (FYI, the number of crumpled tissues scattered around lovers is their way of letting you know how many times they've made love.) Here are some other ways you can stimulate your sense of the visual:

- change the angle of your bed so that you have a different view of the room

- change the lightbulb in your bedside lamp to a different color

- put a colored scarf over the lampshade to give your room an afterglow effect

- move the artwork around on the walls of your room or home

- strategically place a wardrobe mirror so you can watch yourselves

- if you have the space, place a Japanese screen near your bedside, creating a sense of isolation and comfort for you and your lover

207. Pique Your Sense of Hearing.

Seduction begins between your ears, especially for women. Whether you are used to listening to music—soft, hard, or somewhere in the middle—or you enjoy the background vibrations of meditative chants, aural stimulation can offer a deep relaxation that can lead to Great Sex. For some couples, the sound of birds singing through an open window or the eternal sound of a waterfall create a romantic and sensual environment that acts as a passageway to sex. Of course, what you choose to use as such a stimulant or relaxant is purely subjective. But it remains up to you to explore your options.

208. Great Lover Moment: Music to Make Love By.

Whether you are in the mood for hot fast sex, slow romantic sex, or the intensity of some kind of Tantric sex, a recent seminar attendee made these suggestions for music to make love by:

- **Hot Fast Sex:** Try Portishead, Maxwell Urban Suite—or anything with a tribal drumbeat, like reggae.

- **Slow Romantic Sex:** Chet Baker *Songs for Lovers,* Marvin Gaye's "I Want You," Sade's *Deluxe*, John Coltrane's *Coltrane for Lovers,* or Norah Jones's *Come Away with Me*

- **Intense or Inspirational Sex:** Try Margot Anand's "Sky Dancing Tantra: A Call to Bliss," or Joao Gilberto's *Bossa Nova* album.

209. Touch Sensation.

Often men and women have intense sensual memories of how they were touched as babies or children. One man remembers how his grandmother made little circles on his forehead with her fingers. To this day, he melts in response to this kind of touching. A woman from one of my seminars loves her partner to place his hand firmly but gently across the back of her neck. "It soothes and relaxes me instantly." And another man described how intensely his touch connected him to his lover in this way: "It was like her skin was speaking to me." So although we've already discussed the power of touch, I wanted to repeat the message in a slightly different way here. Try these various types of touch:

- short, feathery strokes

- long, irregular swirls

- deep, massaging touch

- then ask what his or her preference is

Next time you're wondering how you might stimulate your lover with touch, ask his or her mother, sister, or grandmother how your lover liked to be touched as he or she went to sleep at night. And also keep in mind that any time you touch someone differently, it will register more intensely since they've never felt it before in quite that way. Need I say more? So ladies and gentlemen, touch your lover everywhere and have his or her skin speak to you.

210. The Swirl.

Here is a tip that men and women love to use to figure out how their lover likes to be touched; it's called the Swirl:

Step One: Using your fingernails, lightly scratch the bare skin of his or her thigh, in a straight line from the knee to the base of the genital area (where the pubic hair begins). Play with the amount of pressure—how does your lover react? Does he or she begin to moan like a cat? Bristle a little? Quiver?

Step Two: Using a big, irregular, wavy motion, go over the same area; this is the Swirl.

Step Three: Continue the swirl over every area of your lover's body—the legs, arms, back, belly, head. And if you really want to rev the engine, do the swirl—albeit lightly and gently—on the genitals.

211. Tantalize Your Sense of Taste.

This tip is related to my suggestions that you dine together often, feed each other often, and explore erotic foods. All of the three former tips have the power to tantalize your taste buds. But the sexual golden ring of taste is, of course, reserved for tasting—and enjoying—each other. I had a man tell me that he found his lover's taste irresistible. "She tastes so good to me, she tastes just right," he said. And because of it he couldn't keep his mouth off of her. Each person has their own distinct, subtle taste. Relish in the taste of your lover.

212. Create a Sanctuary in the Bedroom.

Similar in spirit to the behavior tip Relationship as Refuge, this tip is specific to your bedroom. This is your special room, the place where you and your lover most often come to make love. Therefore, you should give this room an atmosphere that is sensual, comfortable, and has the potential for regular sexual encounters. What style you choose is up to you. Some people are turned on by bedrooms that are pink, white, and frilly. Others prefer the masculine appeal of straight lines and grays and blues and tans. Still others like bedrooms that shine with gold accents. Whatever your preference for interior design, the point is to make sure the room works for the two of you. But there are some things *not* to do:

- don't leave your bed unmade. No one finds used beds appealing, even if it was you who used it

- don't forget to change your sheets regularly

- don't leave your clothes strewn about

- don't fill your room with too much clutter

- don't make the television the room's centerpiece

I rarely like to stress the "Don'ts" of this world, but I feel these reminders are necessary because they all can create obstacles to getting in the mood for Great Sex.

213. Ladies, Prepare the Bed for Your Man with Cool, Crisp Sheets.

Many men have shared with me the divine sensation of slipping into a freshly made bed with crisp, cool linens. Part of this appeal is the feeling of being taken care of, the other part is of a strong, male preference for coolness. I know of one man who so missed the sensation on his cheeks of the cherished coolness of his wife's pressed pillowcases that he shaved his full beard off. Another man said this of slipping into his clean sheets at night, "Once I'm in that bed, she can do anything she wants."

214. Penis Ph.D.

Ladies, you need to study his penis in order to know his penis. Given that your skin is your largest sexual organ, use his penis to your best advantage by acquainting every area of your body with its texture, smell, and feel. As they say about great detectives, leave no stone unturned. Place his penis between your breasts, run your nipple up its silky texture, and even stroke your neck, chin, and nose with it. Use your eyelashes to butterfly kiss the sides of his penis. For those ladies with long hair, wrap a chunk of hair around the shaft to change the texture of your manual stroke. As a good student, you will need to pay close attention to how he reacts and anytime he has an explosive breath, chances are you are doing a very good thing. Instead of using his fingers for manual pleasure, try using his erection to stimulate yourself. Or mount him, lowering your breasts toward his face, and open your genitals with his erect penis.

215. The Penis Effect.

Ladies, use the head of his glans to stimulate yourself clitorally. To do so, straddle him and gently move his penis in contact with your clitoral region. This way he can watch your body and you doing yourself, invariably a truly erotic event for most men.

216. Get to Know Her Essence.

The best way you can be a Great Lover is to open yourself to knowing all of her, so don't be shy, don't be wary. Tell her that you want to know her inside and out. Let her know you think all of her is beautiful. When you look, touch, smell, and kiss her clitoris and the rest of her genitalia, then she will become truly comfortable, and truly yours. Do you really know her genitalia? Do you know exactly how she likes her clitoris stimulated? Do you know where her G spot is located? Use your fingers, mouth, and tongue to investigate her essence. And if you don't know exactly where it is, do some research. The head or glans of the clitoris is just below the place where her inner lips meet at the top. The clitoris is also covered at the top by a small fold of skin called the prepuce. For women who are sensitive to direct clitoral stimulation, this clitoral hood is very protective. And know that just as your penis swells upon stimulation, so too does the clitoral region as it is flooded with blood.

To locate her G spot, put two fingers inside of her vagina and brush them gently through the front, tummy side of the cavity. The G spot swells as it surrounds the urethra and swells, when it is stimulated, in size from a dime to a quarter. And likely I am preaching to the choir when I say her natural scent is what most men say is one of their biggest turn-ons.

217. *Enjoy the Rest of Her Body.*

Once you've become entangled with your lover's genitalia, it's time to shower the rest of her body with your attention. Rub her legs and feet, caress, tickle, gently scratch her arms and hands; kiss, fondle, and mouth her breasts and nipples. Explore her lower back and buttocks—many women love to have this area of their bodies massaged. The key here is to find the areas of her body that she is most proud of or where she is most sensitive and concentrate on them. If you do this in the beginning, you relax her, making it more fruitful to go on to her other areas.

218. *Enjoy the Other Parts of His Body As Well.*

What parts of his body turn you on? Ask yourself these questions as a way to get started. You may know already that you love the small of his back, the inner curve of his arm where it meets his chest. What about his hands, the backs of his legs, the crease where his buttocks and thigh joins? Do you like to tease your fingers through his chest hair? (In my experience, women usually fall into two camps: they either like hair or they don't.) It's up to you to explore and roam. Touch, taste, tickle, inhale: he's offered it all to you. His body is your buffet—it's all yours! And if you are feeling a bit timid or unsure, just ask your lover where you can touch him next—you may never come up for air. Just ask him, "Where to next, darling?" Don't focus on orgasm for the moment, rather, enjoy the texture of his skin, his smell, his very essence. By exploring him in these ways, you will become even closer, more intimate, and connected. As one woman remarked, "When I finally let myself touch my husband in this way, really getting into it, it was like I discovered a whole new world of him. I felt so much closer to him—like we were really one person instead of two." This kind of closeness will make you absolutely present for each other, making you so attuned and engaged that the rest of the world will simply melt away.

219. The Surprise Pleasures of Anal Penetration for Him.

There is a reason why the *Bend Over Boyfriend* video series has been so popular. Simply stated, there are men who want to explore the sensation that women experience when being penetrated by a partner, the sensation of being filled up. Some men know right away that they like or would like to try anal penetration. They are not encumbered by the associations with homosexual sex, may even get off on those associations, or are just born to be more open about their sexuality. Others are more hesitant, so don't push him if he isn't interested. Some men worry that the unwelcome erection they experience during the less than pleasant rectal prostate exam indicated "hidden" tendencies. Actually, congratulations are in order; what is happening is the nerves on either side of the prostate (those responsible for creating your erections) are working just fine. They were simply stimulated during the exam. Also, it stands to reason physically that we would enjoy stimulation of that area, we know how sensitive our lips and mouths are, and that is one end of our GI (gastrointestinal) tract and this is the other end. In any case, if your man is interested in trying anal pleasures, here are a few suggestions:

- Always best after a date-night shower/bidet.

- Lubricate, lubricate, lubricate.

- Start with your finger or fingers and careful of your fingernails.

- Be sure to use a properly designed anal toy, such as an anal plug with a flange (flare) at the base. Begin with smaller toys for insertion and always use plenty of lubrication.

- Try wearing an anal plug during the day to get the area used to sensation. Designer styles are available at www.rosebud.net.

220. Help Her Catch the A-Train.

Gentlemen, if your lady likes to be anally pleasured, or she is interested in trying, she may also like to try what someone dubbed, "Taking the A-Train"—double penetration of her vagina and anus. If you are penetrating her vagina with your penis, you can gently insert your finger, a small dildo, anal plug, or anal beads into her anus. Or if you'd like to be more of a "master of the controls," and don't mind not being inside of her for a moment, then use a dildo vaginally and something smaller (your finger or fingers, anal plug or beads) inside of her anus. And there are novelties designed for double penetration. By gently manipulating both simultaneously, she may leave the station, so to speak—like the A-train.

221. Ladies, Take Charge.

Some men love it when women take charge. So next time you think he may be expecting to see you lying there waiting for missionary style, tell him to lie on his back and then mount him. The sheer momentum you create will have him standing in no time.

222. Have Sex in an Unfamiliar Place.

This tip takes some daring. An unfamiliar place could be anywhere—it really depends on you and what you are used to. If you and your lover typically make love in the bedroom (where 90 percent of sex takes place), then try it in the living room. One couple, Harry and Jill, specialize in finding new or unfamiliar spots, some of which have required a lot of daring and nerve. Consider their choices: the rental storage vault while moving some of her boxes; in the attic of their house while installing insulation; and in a freight elevator—twice in the same night. Most people, however, are more comfortable with the unfamiliar that is still a bit familiar—in the laundry room, for example, or on the washing machine—during the rinse cycle.

223. Have Sex When Others Are Around.

This tip takes even more daring. Another requirement is silence and speed. Consider this scenario: you and your partner are hosting a party. One of you has to go into the garage to replenish the wine or beer supply; the other one follows into the garage. You push the other against the far wall, shimmy your clothes out of the way, and copulate wildly to the sounds of social chitter chatter in the background. At a huge society wedding in Texas, the matron of honor grabbed her tuxedo'd spouse and led him down a secluded hallway of the club so she could give him great oral sex in an unlocked supply cupboard. So perhaps take advantage of a party or occasion at someone else's home. If you and your lover happen to find yourselves in the bathroom at the same time, with the water running, the man can perch the woman on the sink counter and slip her dress up or her jeans down. The man then gets on his knees and gives her oral sex. The danger, the quickness, and the silence come together to give this tip its particular sizzle appeal.

224. Place a Mirror in Your Bedroom.

Why? To watch yourselves having sex of course. This tip came to me from one of my star sex-seminar pupils: She said that when she and her lover added a free-standing dressing mirror, their love nest took on a totally new feeling. And because they could move it, they were able to create new ways of viewing their activities. Indeed, their sex became hotter than ever. So try it, you might like what you see. Men in particular, being visual creatures, really get off on this.

225. Paint Each Other.

There's a particular paint I have in mind—liquid latex body paint—it goes on as easily as it comes off, with soap and water. But the process is absolutely sensational. For the more orally inclined, there are also chocolate body paints, complete with paintbrush and paint. There are also watercolor paint sets that come with their own brushes. Some couples prefer homemade varieties and have been known to get downright creative with peanut butter and honey. Like any artists, you need to follow your instincts and feel free to create, not worrying for the moment about the mess. (You may want to think ahead and put down a big towel as your dropcloth.) Take turns creating watercolors, art, and writing messages on each others' bodies. No only does it feel good, it will also give you both a good laugh and let you explore your creative side. Who knows, your lover may be a latent artist, waiting to emerge!

226. Ask to Be Spanked.

From what I understand, the asking can be as much of a turn-on as the receiving. As one woman said, "One night my husband and I were in the middle of making love, and I just blurted out, 'Spank me!' He looked at me in surprise, but then without a word, he started lightly tapping on my behind. In a few minutes we were both coming. There was something about the illicitness of it that made us both wild."

227. *Give Your Lover a Scalp Massage.*

Most of us love to have our scalps massaged. It's best to do this with dry hair (wet hair has a tendency to pull). And if your partner doesn't mind, put some lotion or light oil on your fingertips as you make light, circular motions around the scalp, paying close attention to cover all territory to move from the base of the neck to the top of the forehead.

228. *Give Your Lover a Back Massage.*

We hold most of our body's tension in our back, which is why so many people are prone to lower-back pain. Have your lover lie on his or her tummy and begin to massage from just above the sacrum (tailbone). Using the sacrum as your center, move outward—up the spine and outward toward the ribs. Massage the upper back and shoulders last, being careful to test how much pressure to use. Make sure you don't put any pressure directly on the spinal cord. Also, warm your hands by rubbing them together first and use a light oil to make your touch more fluid and soothing. There are many massage oils on the market—find one that has the added benefit of aromatherapy. One client found a massage oil called Roman Orgy Love Oil. When he breaks out the bottle, his wife knows she's in for a treat. And its unique scent turns them both on.

229. *Know How to Wash and Brush Your Lover's Hair.*

Gentlemen, most women love to have their hair washed—why do you think they get their hair done at the salon so often? So make a spa date, and wash her hair for her. Whether she's sitting in the kitchen or in the bath or shower, she will love to have your big hands in her hair, massaging in the fragrant shampoo.

Once you're done with the shampoo, comb and brush her hair. If more people only knew how divine it is to have one's hair played with, I would venture to say they would take lessons in brushing their lover's hair. The divine-ness stems from a very simple tenet: Most people have loving, sensual memories of having their hair brushed by their mother or father. Of course, at that time, they didn't think of it as relaxing; they just knew it felt great and wanted more. Now as adults we can ask for more. And any lover worth his or her salt knows relaxation opens the doors to you and your partner being connected.

230. Great Lover Moment: The Magic of a Box of Sand.

One couple recently received a gift that has added a special playfulness to their already stellar love life. The gift was a Japanese meditation box, which looks like a small sandbox, filled with sand and accompanied by a pencillike instrument with which to play in the sand. After receiving the delightful little box, Ann and Chris moved it around their home from room to room, trying to find its perfect place. Finally it landed in their master bathroom, where it has taken on a whole new meaning: When each of them gets up in the morning, they draw or write a message to the other in the sand about how they feel or what they want to do with each other later that day or night. As Ann explained, "We're both such terrible artists that half the fun is about trying to guess what the other one drew!"

231. Shave Him.

Slip into your most sexy lingerie and ask your man to sit down. Then sit astride him (make sure the chair is sturdy) and begin to shave him. Make sure you have all the necessary equipment (warm water, sharp or new razor, his favorite shaving cream, and a hand towel). The mixture of danger and taking care of him is intoxicating. And he will love it.

232. Shave Her Wherever She Wishes.

Whether it is a once-in-a-lifetime gesture or his favorite thing to do in the shower, when your man does this "take-care-of-you" move the memory remains all day long—especially when you cross your legs. As one man said, "Hey, I can't think of anything better than getting to play with her warm wet body first thing in the morning." The beauty of shaving is most men have an awareness of how to warm up the skin, lather the surface and stroke technique, and with that skill set in place he can artfully remove hair from legs and or any other area under your guidance.

233. How to Use Lubricant and Why.

Lubricants have two star qualities: They enhance your sexual pleasure by keeping you both juiced up, and they add a wonderful element of fun to sex. But there are many lubricants to choose from and some that are better for oral sex, others which are better for manual sex, and still others that are best for intercourse and toys. Here is some basic information:

- Use a clear lubricant so you don't worry about staining the sheets.

- Use water-based lubricants. Those that are oil-based will break down the latex of a condom. Also, oil introduced into the vagina can lead to yeast and vaginal infections.

- Make sure the lubricant does not contain the spermicide Nonoxynol-9, which is a harmful irritant to both men and women. This ingredient is also found on some condoms and will take away pleasure, rather than add to it.

234. Coitus Cloths.

Leave a washcloth near the bed. An invaluable research assistant shared this tip with me, referring to her bedside washcloths as "coitus cloths." I rather like that nomenclature. This is, again, a practical tip for cleaning up leaky fluids quickly, without breaking the mood or momentum of the moment, and they are more effective than tissues. Placing them nearby also allows you to linger in bed, rather than jumping up to clean up in the bathroom. They also are particularly handy for those women who prefer not to swallow when giving their men oral sex. My research assistant also suggested that you make any such cloths distinct in color or design from those you use on the rest of your bodies, faces included. This way, you can sort them easily when laundry is done.

235. Keep Your Sex Life Private.

I probably don't have to tell you about this tip, but I will err on the side of caution, and manners. Even though you may sometimes have the urge to share or reveal the intimate details of your relationship to friends or family, just know that one small detail can lead to many broad assumptions. The sex you have with your partner is meant to be private; it's about the two of you and no one else. Once shared, you not only lessen its specialness, but you also risk breaking the bubble of intimacy your relationship is founded upon. So don't tell your friends about how she moans, or about the freckle on his penis. Cherish those details and keep them to yourself.

236. Let Sex Be Fun.

If we can learn to laugh at ourselves in the bedroom, as in any room in our house of life, we eliminate the risk of taking our selves and the situation too seriously. When you laugh and have fun, you avoid giving in to ubiquitous performance pressure. There is a time for hot, steamy, earnest sex, but there are also times when you need to let go and laugh. Sex should be fun. From a certain Luis recounting how he fell out of bed during vigorous activity, to couples cracking up due to someone's "love farts," many couples have shared that some of their best sex has been some of their funniest. Simply said, if you want it to be fun, it will be fun.

The Classics:
Moves, Positions, and More from My Archives

In the Playbook, you learned more than a hundred tips and techniques to keep the fire between you and your lover burning all through late spring and summer. And just when you think you might be due a late-summer break, I want to give you some more very special tips that will turn your fall into an Indian summer, keeping you blazing away. Just like the heading indicates, this section is a collection of the classic moves, positions, and other pointers culled from the archives of my sexuality seminars. Seminar favorites include, Ode to Bryan (perhaps the best manual move on a man), the Ten Ways Women Can Be Stimulated for Orgasm, tips on how to give the best oral sex to a man or a woman, and much, much more. Why are they classics? Because they work and work beautifully and continue to work for many, many people. In the ten years that I've been giving sexuality seminars, I have listened to thousands of women and men tell me what works for them sexually. I have taken this information, added my own ideas, and come up with the best-of-the-best techniques for manual sex, oral sex, inter-course, and anal sex. I've also included tips on developing the spiritual side of sex, as well as particular exercises for increasing your arousal and response factor. So, here is to increasing your sexual pleasure, expanding your sexual knowledge base, and becoming the Great Lover you are no doubt destined to be.

237. Ode to Bryan.

This tip is the all-out favorite hand maneuver for men. A good manual maneuver is an incredibly easy skill to master, and there is one in particular that is a hands-down favorite—no pun intended—The Ode to Bryan. I learned this technique from one of my best male friends who happily taught me this skill using a spoon from a caffe latte. To get ready, position yourself comfortably between his legs. He can sit on a chair, on the edge of the bed, on a stair, or in the back of a taxi. This hand maneuver travels well. Keep in mind that you will be using both of your hands; using both expands the area of sensation and keeps a nice rhythm going.

Step 1: Using your favorite lubricant, apply to the palms of both hands and rub your hands together to warm them and the lubricant.

Step 2: (Illus. 12) You are going to be using both hands, so whichever one you want to start with, place it thumb down, nestled into his pubic hair, palm facing away from you and gently wrap your warmed-up fingers around the base of his penis. "Break" the joint of your wrist and push your wrist toward his stomach so you should now be looking at the back of your hand and four fingers. He should be looking at your thumb. The end of your thumb should rest on the top of your fingertips. Now move your hand up the penis—gently and firmly.

Step 3: (Illus. 13) Only when you get to the top do you release the flexion of your wrist.

Step 4: (Illus. 14) Rotate the palm of your hand over the head of the glans, as if you were caressing the head of a small baby, and drop your fingers so that they are parallel with the shaft so you can maintain palm contact as you rotate over the glans. Bryan's comment was, "The twist is the most crucial part and must be done only at the top. And you

Ode to Bryan

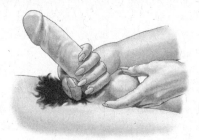

Ill. 12 *Step 2*

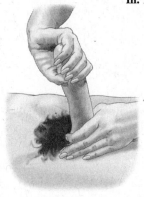

Ill. 13 *Step 3*

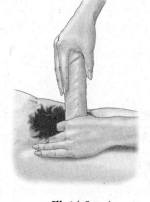

Ill. 14 *Step 4*

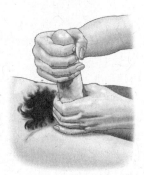

Ill. 15 *Step 5a*

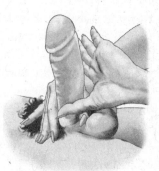

Ill. 16 *Step 6*

must keep as much of your hand as possible in contact with the penis at all times to create maximum sensation and stimulation."

Step 5a: (Illus. 15) Once your hand has rotated over, and keeping the palm in contact, flip your hand so that you have a little ring with the index finger and forefinger.

Step 5b: Complete that hand's stroke by continuing to the bottom of his shaft.

Step 6: (Illus. 16) Just as you complete the one hand's cycle, your other hand should already be in position at the base to start the upward stroke.

Step 7: Repeat as needed . . .

238. *It Takes Three.*

Most women love to be manually stimulated; indeed, since their first orgasm usually happens through masturbation, many women are able to orgasm easily and intensely this way. Before getting started, do two things: 1) clean and warm your hands; 2) apply lubricant (water based). And keep this general tip in mind: When touching a woman's genitals, always begin with broad strokes, reducing the area of stimulation as sensation builds. Here's a favorite hand maneuver—It Takes Three.

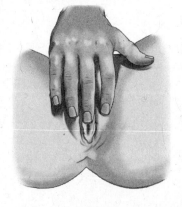

Step 1) Using your three middle fingers, as seen in **illustration 17,** curve them over her vulva, warming the area and getting her ready for touching so that no one area, especially the clitoris, is shocked—not exactly a turn-on. Using your middle finger, gently finger her clitoral area and the bud.

Ill. 17 *Step 1*

Step 2) Maintain a slow up-and-down motion while slowly slipping your middle finger into her vagina **(illustration 18).**

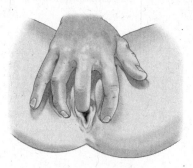

Ill. 18 *Step 2*

Step 3) Finally, with your middle and index fingers together, as in **illustration 19,** stimulate the clitoral ridge with a up-and-down motion. Some women like to have the bud squeezed gently; others prefer a pulsing sensation; still others want the continued up-and-down motion of your fingers.

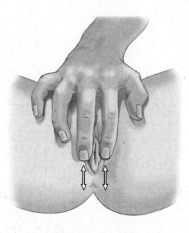

Ill. 19 *Step 3*

You may want to consider **(illustration 20)** as it is what some Great Lovers have said is their preferred way to do It Takes Three and The Y-Knot, which follows. This position allows the woman to relax mentally into the sensations while remaining physically completely connected to her man.

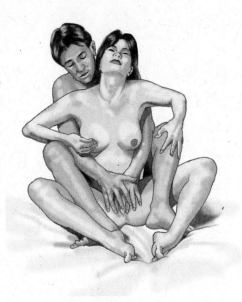

Ill. 20

239. Y-Knot.

This is another manual maneuver a man can do on his lady. The basic move is to spread open her lips with one hand, while massaging her clitoris with the other hand. As the illustration suggests, use two fingers on one hand for spreading, and the middle finger of your other hand for a circular or up-and-down motion. And if she enjoys it, slip your middle finger inside of her every once in a while. Remember to keep the delicate vulva tissue moist to ease motion and so that it doesn't start to dry out and feel uncomfortable.

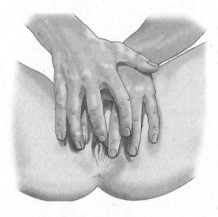

Ill. 21

240. Basket Weave.

A favorite of seminar attendees and their men.

Step 1: With well-lubricated hands clasp your hands together as seen in **illustration 22** (top view) and lower them over his erect penis.

Step 2: Remember your hands are acting like an imposter vagina so mimic the sensation similar to that of when a man first enters you.

Step 3: Start what will be a continuous up-and-down twisting motion by slowly lowering your hands down his shaft as seen in the side view of **illustration 23.**

Step 4: Illustration 24 shows the gentle rotation you do at the base of his shaft before you start the upward stroke. The twisting motion is done continuously while doing the up-and-down stroke to heighten sensation for him. The motion is like that of a washing machine done very gently.

Basket Weave

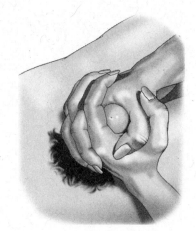

Ill. 22

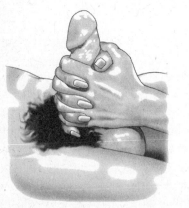

Ill. 23

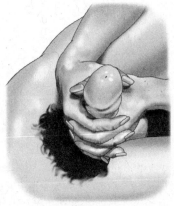

Ill. 24

241. The Art of Giving Her Oral Pleasure.

Most women come alive when they are pleasured orally. It's one of the most intimate, loving acts a man can perform for his woman. Also, for a high percentage of women, this is one of the easiest ways to orgasm. Why? Because of the constant stimulation in combination with the heat, softness, and moisture of your mouth. Men who have the gift of cunnilingus are often referred to as "artists"—because of the attitude with which they pleasure their woman. As any artist will tell you, all art is subjective and personal, and no two women are alike in what they prefer and what they need to enjoy themselves. The male artist in this case prepares his woman's sensation canvas according to her particular needs and desires, and then uses his tools to take her to another level. Gentlemen, use the following tips to guide you as you paint your lover's canvas, but know that without the attitude and intention of pleasing her and her alone, there will be no masterpiece, merely a counterfeit production.

242. Head-On or Profile?

Some women prefer direct stimulation of the clitoris and others find this too intense. And some women change during the course of their monthly hormonal cycles, becoming too sensitive for direct stimulation the middle two weeks of the cycle, when they are most sensitive, and during the rest of the time, absolutely craving direct stimulation. Now, gentlemen, if you are with a lady who loves the intensity of straight-on stimulation, you may want to vary the intensity by lifting the clitoral hood to expose more of the extremely sensitive glans underneath. This is most easily done while you are between her legs and can apply pressure onto her pubic hair. As if you are moving a cheek to make someone smile, gently push the pubis mons toward her tummy. This way more of the inner labia (lips) and clitoris will be available for stimulation. Or, depending on your preferred position, if you are between her legs and lying more horizontally, use your middle and index fingers of both hands to lift the outer labia like small tent poles so that you can explore more of that incredibly soft skin with your mouth. That will be some camping trip.

243. Vary the Speed and Pressure of Your Tongue.

It is the variation of sensation that allows for the greatest buildup of pleasure when you are giving oral sex to a lady. Once you have reached that certain point, you then maintain intensity until completion. The reason you do not use the same strength of touch at the beginning as you do at the end is because those incredibly sensitive nerves need to acclimate to the intensity. If you are too strong or too quick with your tongue, then you may numb her. And like a good dancer, you don't get on the dance floor and use the same step through the whole song; you vary your strokes until the dance is done.

244. For the More Delicate Flowers.

If your lover is too sensitive for direct clitoral stimulation, you may want to consider the following options: 1) Alternate between a broad stroke and a pointy one, circling the clitoral bud, but not stimulating the glans (the most sensitive part) directly. A broad stroke is achieved by flattening out the tip of your tongue; a pointy stroke is when you narrow the tip of your tongue into a point; 2) Have her wear sheer, silk panties and pleasure her through the material. Wet silk adheres very well to any surface and is the perfect governor of intensity for extremely sensitive women. Also, please know that just because a woman is sensitive does not mean it will necessarily be easy to stimulate her. Again, if the pressure is too intense, she can be pushed out of the feel-good realm and into the it-hurts realm. And I can assure you that once something begins to hurt, it's almost impossible to return to feeling good. Rather than take the risk, simply start out more gently and gradually build pressure.

245. The Nose Knows (AKA Face Facts).

Women have long known that it is not an urban myth that men with big noses can provide special sexual satisfaction. A large nose does not promise a larger size "down there," but rather a truer suggestion that men who have been blessed with larger noses often use them very well during oral sex. As one of my suppliers said, "The nose knows." Some men use the rounded end of their nose when their tongues get tired, or simply because they love the sensation of the smooth, buttery texture of her labia and clitoris against their nose. Some men are so turned by their partner's scent, it's as if they want to drink their essence into them. Other men use their chins to create pressure on the bottom of the introitus (the entry into the vagina), while still other men use their pursed lips to open up the labia before sucking them into their mouths.

246. The Kivin Method.

The beauty of the Kivin Method is that you can create intense oral stimulation for a woman while getting immediate feedback that you are in the right place. You can also use this method to add a new angle for both of you. For ease of explanation, locate the K and C points on the diagram. Then follow the directions below:

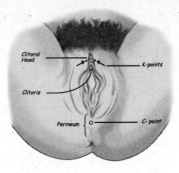

Clitoral
Hood

K-points

Clitoris

Perineum

C- point

Ill. 25

- The man lies perpendicular to the woman at a 90-degree angle to her hip.

- The woman's only responsibility is to receive sensation.

- The partner uses a back-and-forth tongue stroke over the hood of the clitoris. Men who have practiced this technique have said that when the woman is aroused, they can feel two bumps on either side of the clitoral hood that feel like half grains of rice. These are the K points.

- The C point is how to get immediate feedback from the woman that you are in the right place. The man places his middle finger on her perineum, the C point, which is the quarter-size area between the vagina and anus. Make sure your nails are short and that she can only feel your finger pad, not your nail. The reason you will get immediate feedback is when your tongue is stroking in the correct place, the woman will experience involuntary, preorgasmic contractions in this area. Your finger doesn't move; it stays still, because if you do move your finger you may move her concentration from the clitoral hood area to the perineum. By reading her body, you will be able to maintain correct tongue placement without wondering, "Am I there? Where is there? Have I moved from there?"

- Once you have started, don't stop. Continue past her initial orgasmic response, as often this stimulation is the most intense and satisfying portion of the orgasm.

- Some couples have added a position adjustment: The woman curls her legs up to her chest and the man uses his arm to keep them pushed back and stabilized. In this way, the woman is very widely spread open and can receive even more intense stimulation.

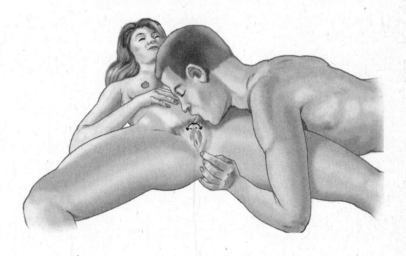

Ill. 26

247. Big, Soft, Wet, and Warm.

Gentlemen, in giving oral sex to a woman, kiss her lips south of the border as you would her upper lips. If you have trouble envisioning how to kiss a woman "down there," just imagine that you are kissing her lips: Both areas respond to heat, moisture, and texture. So kiss her in an all-encompassing manner—big, soft, wet, and warm, and stay in constant contact.

248. *Please, No Flicking.*

My number-one piece of advice for men when giving their ladies oral pleasure: Please don't just flick. As a way to start, flicking may be fine, but be aware that it is a rotten holdover of visual information from the adult industry. If they showed in adult films what really works for most women, you wouldn't see the tongue at all. In other words, the flicking depiction is a way to get a good shot for a film, but not a good way to orally pleasure a woman. Flicking is just like it sounds: short, annoying licks with your tongue against her clitoris or vaginal lips. These strokes make it difficult for women to build up sensation and feel any pleasure at all. The solution? Be aware that women are open to your using your tongue in all sorts of ways: Some women prefer wide, lush strokes. Other women prefer quick, hard strokes with the top of your tongue. Still other women prefer the soft underside of your tongue in a back-and-forth motion over the clitoris, and for some, sucking pulsations over the clitoris do the trick. But I've never heard of a woman who enjoys the flicking depicted in porn films.

249. *A Tip for Sucking Her.*

Many men come to me, asking how they should lick or suck a woman orally. This piece of advice came from one woman who voiced it in a seminar: "Suck on us the way you want us to suck on you." Want to know how? Get guidance from your partner; obviously, this is a two-way street on the preferred level of suction. So, gentlemen, if you know in advance that your lady likes to have you suck on her genitals, then try doing it in the same way you suck on her tongue while French kissing her. Also, ask her if that would feel good elsewhere and if you need to adjust suction. Indeed, the best way to determine how much or little suction she likes is to simply suck on her finger or her tongue and ask if that's her preference—this way she can give you direct feedback.

250. Tips for the Tongue-Tired.

Gentlemen, if your tongue gets tired when you are orally pleasuring her, you can maintain contact and sensation for her while giving yourself a bit of a break without slowing down the pace. Wrap your tongue over your upper lip and use the incredibly soft underside of your tongue to maintain her stimulation. FYI, this underbelly of your tongue has a nifty little ridge that can add to her sensation. You can give your tongue a further break by wagging your head in a "no" motion; this way you don't have to use your tongue, but you are still maintaining contact and giving her the back-and-forth motion that is so crucial for most women. And the added bonus of the "wag" is getting the knots out of your neck.

251. Avoid That Crink in Your Neck.

Gentlemen, this tip is for you when giving your lady oral sex. Grab two pillows and place one under your chest and one under her hips. This way, your chin is not scrunched along the mattress or surface. With her pelvis in a more uplifted position, you now have greater range of motion. Also, in this more elevated position, you can support your chin on your clenched fist with your chin in the circle created by the ring finger and forefinger. Your index finger can also do double duty in this position by perhaps stroking the clitoral area, stroking across her perineum, or, as some women prefer, inserting your finger into her vagina with a pressure down onto the bottom of the introitus (entry into the vagina).

252. School Days—Forming Those Letters.

Gentlemen, most women prefer you to use your tongue in small movements across the clitoris. To make this more than an exercise, and more interesting to you (it's already interesting to her), you can easily create more of a range of motion by writing letters of the alphabet with your tongue—thanks to Sam Kinison for this tip. Then change the font, or compose a sentence. This move should not be confused with flicking because you are using your tongue with steady-but-gentle pressure that allows for sensation to build. The majority of women prefer the slow building of sensation that comes from such repetitive motion. Another tip said to be attributed to Whoopi Goldberg: Cunnilingus aficionados should train by using Lifesavers: place the Lifesaver up against closed teeth and use unique tongue patterns and moves to make the candy dissolve. By studying the surface of the candy with your tongue—the hole, the raised writing, the edges, and the smooth parts—you are getting in great shape for exploring all the sides of a woman. And should you choose to practice this Lifesaver technique on the subway, no one will be the wiser.

253. The Power of Eye Contact.

Ladies, maintain eye contact when giving him oral or manual sex. Remember, men are visual creatures, and want to see you getting turned on while turning them on. So don't hide behind a mask of hair or turn your head away from them. As one representative man said, "When she looks straight into my eyes with my penis in her mouth, it's all I can do not to explode. It's a total turn-on."

254. The Ring and the Seal.

This tip is the key to giving great oral sex to your man. There are basically six components to great oral sex on your man, which I will teach you here. The first two moves are for preparation:

1. Create a RING with your thumb and forefinger while the other fingers mirror the
   shape of the index finger and wrap around
   the penis to create a tunnel.

2. SEAL that RING to your mouth, sort of like a little tube to your
   lips. Basically, you are extending the length of area with which you
   can pleasure your man. Once the RING and the SEAL are in place,
   you're ready for the best oral sex of his life.

      Keep in mind that there are three things that men say ab-
   solutely make entering a woman during sex so incredible: the combination of heat, pressure, and moisture. So in essence, with your
   hand "sealed" to your mouth, you are creating a pseudo-vagina
   with your hand and mouth. The beauty of this move is that your
   hand supplies the pressure, so no more bruises and teeth-marked
   inner lips, and no more sore jaw muscles from trying to create pressure while covering your teeth, the RING does that for you. The
   RING and SEAL do not separate.

3. Up/down. With your RING sealed to your mouth, which delivers the heat and moisture, establish a comfortable grip on his erect shaft and proceed to move in a continuous up-and-down motion along the length to create stimulation;

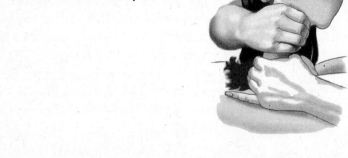

4. Twisting. At the same time, imagine the RING SEALED to the outside of your lips to be on ball bearings—made much easier if there is plenty of saliva or a lubricant of your choice—continuously and gently rotate your hand (remember, it's sealed to your mouth);

5. Tongue in motion. At the same time, about a half inch of your tongue will extend into the notch between your index finger and thumb so that you can use the tastebud surface to maintain a hot/warm back-and-forth stroke across the frenulum (that is the V-shaped area at the head of the penis on the underside);

6. And you will also be creating sensation in expanded areas away from the penis itself. With your free hand, stimulate another part of his body, inside of the thighs, nipples—and don't forget his testicles—just remember to treat them like small, breakable eggs and you will be fine. Also, some men use a firm, stroking motion on their lower abdomen with their free hand when masturbating; you can mimic this while doing things orally to him by using the side of your hand like a little squeegee, making a firm stroke from the belly button area down toward the base of the shaft. Other options are to stroke across the perineum under the scrotum with your thumb. Watch your nails or bend your index and middle fingers; also use your smooth-knuckle area in a circular motion here.

255. Don't Forget to Mind the Stepchildren.

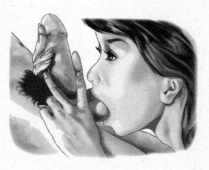

To what am I referring here? Your man's testicles. Why the name? During a ladies' seminar, when we were discussing how a man's testicles and scrotum are often overlooked (because so much of our attention is focused on the penis), a woman with a thick Texan accent announced, "Omigod, they are being treated like stepchildren; they are being totally ignored!" I thought I'd die laughing—even though I've been both a stepchild and a stepmother myself, and do not think this term is at all derogatory. But truly, ladies, more men want this tender area played with than they do their bottoms. The small, breakable egg rule applies here unless you are instructed to handle them otherwise. Some men want them sucked, some held, and some cupped by a hand up against the body. Some men like you to hold the scrotum, the bag they are in, away from the body by making a small circle with the index finger and thumb and gently stretching the skin away. Other men prefer the "take it home" move: when a woman uses a "come here" stroking motion with all her fingers underneath the scrotum.

256. Ladies, Strum the Frenulum.

A man's frenulum is the quarter-size area at the underside of his penis. Most women refer to this place as the "V." The word "frenulum" actually means mucous membrane attachment point, and for most men this area of nerve endings is a hotspot. It is more obvious on circumcised men, but equally, if not more so, as sensitive for uncircumcised men. When a woman strokes or sucks on it—using either her mouth, tongue, or fingers—she elicits tremendous and often intense sensation.

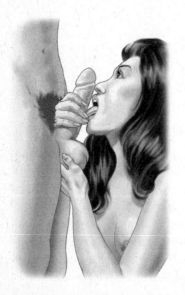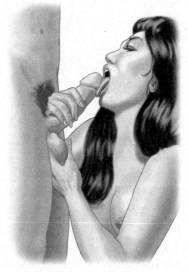

Ill. 31

So ladies, when you happen to be hovering in the general vicinity, remember to pay attention to this sensational area of his anatomy. But keep in mind that like your clitoris, this area can get overstimulated, so do not concentrate too long in one spot as you may numb him by being too intense, unless of course he asks for it.

257. The Ten Ways Women Can Be Stimulated to Achieve Orgasm.

Women can achieve orgasm in many different ways, specifically ten. The ten "operative ways" described in the tips below demonstrate the range of female sexual sensitivity—so next time you are roaming her body, just keep in mind that there is a possibility that you may induce an orgasm at any moment.

258. #1 CLITORAL

The most common form of orgasm for women, the clitoral orgasm, can happen through manual stimulation, oral stimulation, his penis (massaging against her clitoral area), his thigh, or by stimulation of toys such as dildos, or vibrators. Women describe this orgasmic sensation as a pulling-up-and-into the body. The nerve system being stimulated is the pudendal.

259. #2 VAGINAL AND CERVICAL

This type of orgasm is stimulated by deep pressure and stimulation within the vagina, or on the cervical area, usually through the in-and-out motion of the penis during intercourse or a toy. The nerve system involved is the pelvic/hypogastric, and women describe the sensation from stimulation of this area as a more all-over-body sensation and similar to a "bearing down" at the point of orgasm.

260. #3 G spot and AFE (anterior fornix erotic) Zone

The G spot is so-named because of a small, roundish tissue area felt through the lining of the front, or tummy, side of the vaginal wall, past the pubic bone. Some women can experience powerful orgasms through the manual or penile stimulation of this area. In the Playbook, you will find a GLM in which I present the step-by-step instructions used by Dr. Beverly Whipple (the researcher who named the G spot) for a woman to find her own G spot . . . should she wish to. But let's not make it the sexual Holy Grail. For some women, the G spot orgasm is the Bomb, for others, stimulating this area does

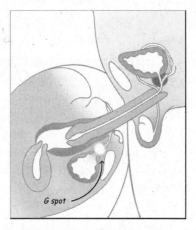

(stimulation during rear entry intercourse)

nothing. The AFE zone is also located inside the vagina, but farther up the vaginal vault, nearer to the cervix. Different from the G spot, which usually requires steady and firm stroking to lead to climax, the AFE is most effectively stimulated through quick, light strokes on the tummy side of the vaginal wall.

261. #4 Urethral (u-spot)

Located between the clitoral glans and the vaginal opening, the urethra is the place where urine exits the body. Some women can experience powerful orgasms with firm manual or oral pressure on this area and for some during intercourse (female-superior position 33 C). The reason for that is so physiologically simple: The urethra is surrounded on three sides by the body of the clitoris.

262. #5 BREAST/NIPPLE

Some women love to have their breasts and nipples fondled; others don't. But for those who enjoy having their breasts and nipples stimulated, intense sensations can be created from light licking and hot breath all the way through to the intensity of firm pinching and nipple clips. Indeed, renowned sexologist and therapist Herbert A. Otto, Ph.D, claims in his book, *Liberated Orgasm*, that the breast/nipple orgasm is actually the second most common form of orgasm for women and the most common when seriously heavy petting was the norm before birth control was readily available.

263. #6 MOUTH

Unusual, but not impossible, this particular source of orgasm begins with the lips and radiates outward through the mouth, tongue, and down the throat. Like the breast/nipple orgasm, the mouth orgasm is more commonly reported when couples have extended heavy petting and kissing sessions.

264. #7 ANAL

Those who are comfortable with anal play are probably already familiar with how intense anal stimulation and anal orgasm can be—for either men or women. This type of stimulation can be done with the mouth (analingus), in which the tongue strokes around the rectum area, or through the insertion of fingers (watch your nails), toys, or penis. One analingus technique in particular is called Rose Petals, in which you move your tongue in tiny circular loops, as if you are tracing the sepals (the small green leaves at the bottom) of a rose, and then move your tongue in a circle around the rim of the anus (this is known as rimming).

265. #8 Blended/Fusion

This type of orgasm comes about when more than one area of the body becomes stimulated and then aroused at the same time. It's common, for example, for a woman to experience a clitoral orgasm and a vaginal at the same time, and that is because the two separate sexual nerve systems are being stimulated at the same time, the pudendal (clitoral) and the pelvic/hypogastric (G spot). Men, too, have these two nerve systems pudendal (penis) and the pelvic/hypogastric (prostate).

266. #9 Zone

This particular form of orgasm is one that occurs when an area not typically considered erotic or associated with the erogenous zones of the body becomes excited. If a woman becomes excited to the point of orgasm when her thighs are massaged, or feet rubbed, then they have experienced a zone orgasm. Men too have had orgasms from, as an example, having the sides of their necks rubbed.

267. #10 Fantasy

Just like it sounds, this form of orgasm occurs when some women (and men, too) can experience an orgasm through a visual or aural fantasy, using only their minds with no touching of their bodies.

268. *Great Lover Moment: Cinematographers Rule.*

I'm speaking of one cinematographer in particular, who told me about a wonderful way to give his lady a urethral orgasm during oral sex. During oral sex, while he is moving his tongue back and forth on her clitoris, he wraps his lower lip over his bottom teeth and presses up firmly onto the urethral glans. Since the urethra is surrounded on three sides by the clitoris, this pressure on the urethral area gives the clitoral region intense stimulation. Gentlemen, try a gentle up-and-down motion with your lip as you maintain pressure. Be sure to shave closely before doing this, so she won't feel the stubble.

269. *The Fab Four of Male Orgasm.*

As to be expected, men and women experience orgasms differently. In general, men orgasm in four different places:

1. in the penis (usually accompanied by ejaculation)

2. in the prostate or anus

3. in the nipples

4. in the mouth from kissing

270. *The Eight Ways Men Orgasm.*

Similar to women, men can elicit an orgasm in numerous ways—eight to be exact.

1. Through intercourse

2. Through manual stimulation of the penis

3. Through oral stimulation of his genitals

4. Through stimulation of his prostate and/or anus

5. Stimulation of his nipples/breast

6. Blended, in which two areas are stimulated at once

7. Through mental stimulation or fantasy

8. Zone orgasm—two or more places at once

271. Anal Play—Debunking the Myths.

In my sexuality seminars, I am often asked to give my opinion of anal sex, and I respond that if anal sex gives you pleasure, then by all means, cede to and enjoy that pleasure. But for those of you who may remain a bit uncomfortable or who have questions about anal sex, I refer you to two books Tristan Taormino's *The Ultimate Guide to Anal Sex for Women* and Jack Morin's *Anal Pleasure & Health: A Guide for Men and Women*. Ms. Taormino points out ten myths about anal sex. When giving your man or your lady anal pleasure, it's important to be aware that these ten ideas are false (and I quote directly):

1. anal sex is unnatural and immoral

2. only sluts, perverts, and weirdoes have anal sex

3. the anus and rectum were never meant to be eroticized

4. anal sex is dirty and messy

5. only homosexual men have anal sex

6. straight men who like anal sex are really gay

7. anal sex is always painful for the person on the receiving end

8. women don't enjoy receiving anal sex; they do it just to please their partners

9. anal sex is the easiest way to get AIDS

10. anal sex is naughty

Recently, there has been more anal sex shown in adult male porn; as a result, more men have been requesting to sample this pleasure with their ladies. Both of you need to feel comfortable with this request: remember, it's up to you. For some people, anal play is the best thing they ever discovered, and for others, it is simply not an option. Your choice. The next few tips give you some added information about how to increase your pleasure during anal sex.

272. Cleanliness Is Next to Godliness.

If you and your man enjoy anal stimulation, then it's absolutely crucial that everything involved be clean: hands, anus/rectum area, and any toys. Wash all such equipment with antibacterial soap, and keep any anal toys separate from those that may be used vaginally. This is one time your mother was wrong about sharing: Your toys are to be used on you alone.

273. Relax.

It's also important for you to relax the anal area as much as possible. What we do not get told clearly is the fact that there are two sphincters (muscle rings) in the anus: one is under voluntary control, and the other is under involuntary control. The first you can relax just by thinking about doing so; but the second requires that you use a finger or a toy to relax and dilate the opening so that penetration is a pleasurable experience. Try warming up the area by gently inserting your well-lubricated finger (or fingers) with only water-based lubrication into your lover's anus before penetration. And use the following rule: one finger for one minute, two fingers for two minutes.

274. Around the Globe.

This tip will provide you with a global view of the six positions for intercourse. Although you may have heard that there are hundreds of positions for intercourse, there really are only six basic positions and everything else is a variation on a theme of those positions. Within these six basic positions are a multitude of options to create variety for whatever mood you and your partner may be in. Some couples like to try several positions during one lovemaking encounter—indeed, 2–3 positions is the average for each lovemaking session. As the accompanying illustrations indicate, there are several variations for each position. I suggest that you and your partner take a look at these together—not so much to memorize the positions and their variations (trust me, once you look at them, the information is stored in your brain), but to stir your appetite for variation itself. So, for your pleasure, here are the six basic positions.

275. #1 Female Superior

In this position, the woman is on top of the man. The degree of her angle (whether she is seated and vertical or more horizontal), will affect how much stimulation she creates for herself and her partner as it is the woman who controls the motion and amount of sensation. In **illustration 33a,** a woman can enhance her own G spot stimulation by arching her back during her vertical motions.

Some couples enjoy the teasing nature of **illustration 33b.** In this position the head of the man's glans is kept right at the entry of the introitus, vaginal entry, for maximum sensation for both. The completion of this is often a firm downward stroke where the woman takes the entire length of the shaft inside of her after having highly aroused him. The woman may be either facing him or facing away. **Illustration 33c** shows a preferred position for women who enjoy strong urethral stimulation. And for those ladies who know their partners enjoy a rear view that combines strong glans stimulation, **33d** is for them. She controls what works for her, while providing his desired scenery. The feet on the bed allows more vertical motion than just being on your knees, and he supports her with his arms.

Ladies, as you have seen, some men love when they have a view of their lovers' derrieres; other men like watching their lovers' faces as they move up and down. And some men get totally jazzed when women lower themselves onto them, starting at the top of the head, and moving down the body slowly. Of course, variety is the spice of life, so alternating is probably best. So, ladies, inquire and inspire.

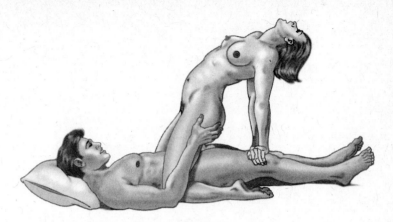

Ill. 33a

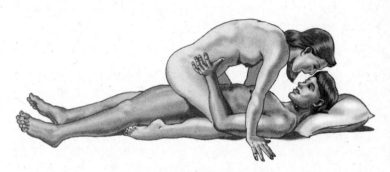

Ill. 33b

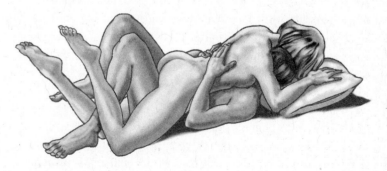

Ill. 33c

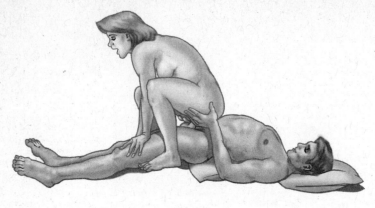

Ill. 33d

276. #2 Male Superior

The man is on top in this position, AKA missionary style. Probably the most popular, it is also a favorite because it encourages kissing, caressing, and other forms of interaction between the two of you. Hence, it tends to be the most romantic. And contrary to what many may think, women don't have to be passive in this position: They can remain quite active. Consider these two options: once the man has entered, you bend your knees and plant your feet on the bed/floor/surface and use the strength of your thighs and hip flexors to create the sensations you want. And you can also use your hands to fondle his testicles as seen in **illustration 34a** or insert a finger in his anus.

In **illustration 34b,** the important part of his body placement is how high up he is on the woman's body. Use of a strong hip curl means that he will be in constant contact with her clitoral area. And in this position, the woman can also guide his angle by pulling him up her body with her arms.

For tighter clitoral stimulation, see the position illustrated by **34c.** The man has entered the woman and then she closes her legs and his legs go to the outside. This enhances two things: more total-body contact and an increase in the tightness of entry. Look at the feet as well. By using her feet as a brace for motion, the man can maintain much more effective clitoral stimulation with shorter strokes instead of the longer in and out of usual male-superior intercourse. Other orgasms that can be achieved in this position are the urethral and vaginal/cervical.

Position **34d** shows how a man can control the angle of his penis inside of the woman to stimulate her G spot, while she can adjust the tilt of her pelvis to the desired angle.

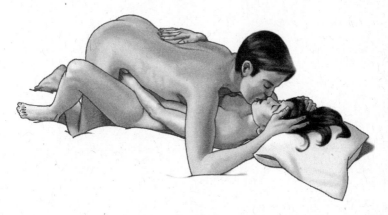

Ill. 34a

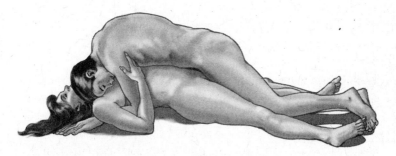

Ill. 34b

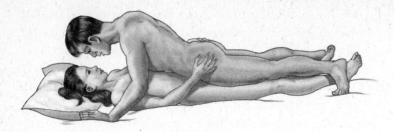

Ill. 34c

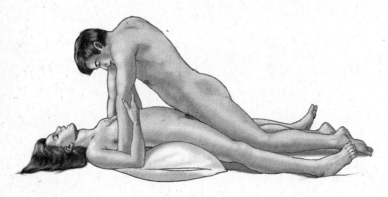

Ill. 34d

277. #3 Side by Side

In this position, the man and the woman lay side by side, either facing each other or with one behind (usually the man, for obvious reasons). This position is warm and comforting rather than high energy. Spooning is a position many couples like to fall asleep in. And should the mood move them, side by side is also good for Middle of the Night Sex (see **illustration 11, page 138**). Some women don't like this position because there is less penetration; but men prefer it because they usually last longer before coming. When the man is behind the woman, while he is inside of her, he can gently fondle her genitals as seen in **illustration 35a.** Women love this double sensation on the clitoris and inside, filling them up. Should you want to explore G spot stimulation in this position, look at **illustration 35b.** By using the combined strength of

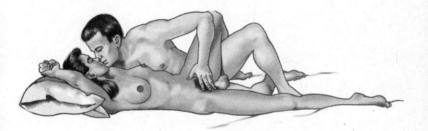

Ill. 35a

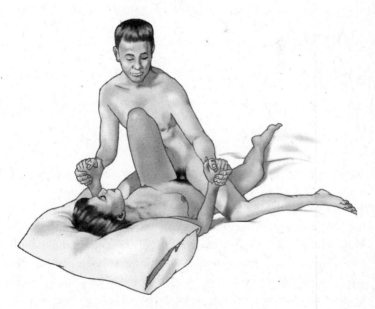

Ill. 35b

your arms, you can easily adjust your angle and depth of penetration. And for those who are not questing for the G spot, this is a variety favorite to add to their options. **Illustration 35c** is a Great Lover favorite for post-coital glow. You can easily rest and still maintain maximum connection.

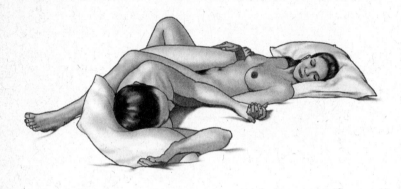

Ill. 35c

278. #4 Rear Entry—AKA Doggie Style

In this position, the man enters the woman from behind—from either a kneeling or standing position. This position **(illustration 36a)** allows a man the deepest level of penetration, and as a result, it is a very popular among women, especially those who enjoy G spot stimulation. And women who have delivered vaginally have a better ability to orgasm from G spot stimulation in this position. Why? Because the vagina is more flexible post-delivery, so the head of his glans will stroke firmly over the appointed spot more easily. And the woman can vary both the G spot and depth of penetration intensity of this stroke merely by raising or lowering her shoulders. Some Great Lovers find this to be one of their hottest fantasy positions. Many men love this position for quick, passionate, high-energy sex—why? Because of the intense glans stimulation, they tend to come very quickly! I've also been told by my field researchers that some men love the intensity of the smell of sex when making love in this position. Men also say they like this position because they can feel their thighs slapping up against the back of hers. Oh, and did I mention they love the more animal nature of this? The only caveat for men on this position is to not to have so much "swing" they make their scrotums sore. For those who prefer rear entry with less motion, **36b** illustrates a seated option—one many have used to advantage thanks to large skirts, and in spas.

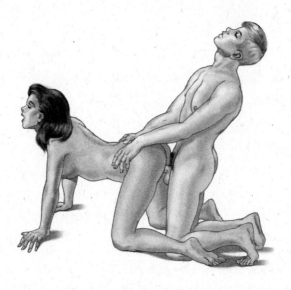

Ill. 36a

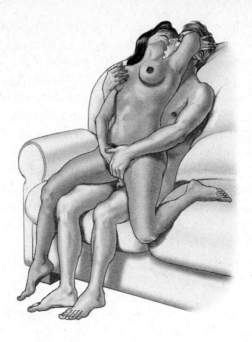

Ill. 36b

279. #5 Sitting/Kneeling

This position is similar to female superior because the woman sits or kneels atop the man. This is a great position for when a woman is pregnant because there is less penetration, and the position directs the penis to the vaginal roof (as seen in **illustration 37a**) instead of putting pressure on the back of her cervix. But it's also a great transition position—for those couples who like to vary their positions throughout a lovemaking session—which is just about all of us. A woman can also have a clitoral orgasm quite easily in this position—through manual stimulation by her lover or herself—as he is penetrating her. Some women also find they can come vaginally by adjusting the thrusting motion. In **illustration 37b,** you can see a creative way for the woman to use the strength of his thighs to control motion while giving herself firm vertical motion.

The Better Than Sex position **(illustration 37c)** is a favorite for intense stimulation for both partners. This is also a great position for strong stimulation of the G spot front vaginal wall from his penis, as well as very strong glans stimulation for him due to the angle of entry into her vagina. Other plusses of this position include making it easier for the woman to go into her own space by closing her eyes while stimulating herself with her own hand on her clitoris, and the man's additional bonus of seeing her breasts move with his thrusts and watching her face get flushed with the sensation. Also, he can show off all the work he has done at the gym by flexing and showing her his "Big Guns" in action.

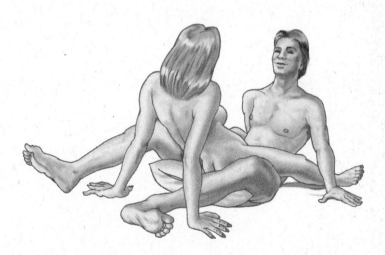

Ill. 37a

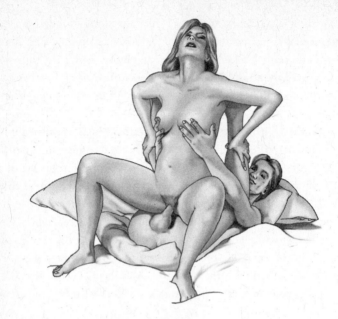

Ill. 37b

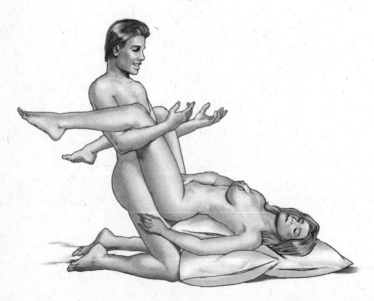

Ill. 37c

280. #6 Standing

I would advise couples not to do this position without support—a wall, a chair, against the bed. While I trust you are all well balanced, this position may challenge the best of you. The Standing position packs a powerful punch because you have more overall muscular contractions throughout your entire body, which in turn enhances the sexual response. This tip comes from my Russian tailor: When having sex on stairs, as seen in **illustration 38a,** have the woman stand on the upper step and place one leg over the railing and then the man can enter her and they both can maintain motion and balance by holding the railing. He can also hold on to her garter belt—see, they do have a function after all. Should you choose to do things from behind, say on a balcony while watching the sunset, option **38b** would be your likely choice.

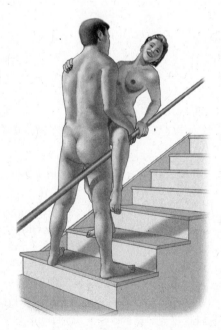

Ill. 38a

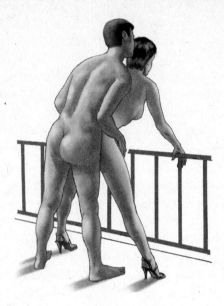

Ill. 38b

281. Great Lover Moment: Be Your Own Judge of Arousal.

One woman in a sexuality seminar made an important point about the pressure some women feel to become aroused. As she put it, "Men have erections to show their arousal, but what do we have to show? Erect nipples and a budding clitoris? I don't think so." My advice, ladies, is to be calm and sure about your own arousal. Don't think it has to show. Typically, he will know you are aroused by a combination of the changes in your breathing rate and your lubrication.

282. Mindful Breathing Techniques That Enhance Sexual Experience.

It's all in the breath. You've all probably heard this advice before. But when it comes to sex, learning how to breathe more consciously has tremendous power to not only enhance overall body stimulation, but also extend orgasm. This is a simple but powerful technique to use during sensation buildup, near the point of orgasm, or both. Some couples practice first while self-pleasuring to get acquainted with the body sensations:

- **Step One**—hold your breath and note the sensation, then do regular deep breaths and see how the sensations expand and deepen

- **Step Two**—continue with regular deep breaths

- **Step Three**—as you wish to increase the sensation, start panting just before orgasm and feel these panting sensations expand throughout your entire body and fill your head

283. Exploring the Yoni and Lingam—Tantric Techniques of Sexual Pleasure.

There has been a lot written about, spoken about, and advertised about Tantric sex, much of it less than accurate, less than helpful, or both. Essentially, Tantric sex is an expanded form of yoga used by a couple to achieve spiritual enlightenment. In sexual terms, the most primary intention is to connect more deeply and not to rush to mere orgasmic gratification. In Tantra one delays orgasm as long as possible in order to open up the body, and thereby the soul, to allow for as much sensation as possible. When the body is so open, you are then better able to experience a union that is both spiritual and sexual with your mate. By opening your bodies, as a couple, to this degree and breadth of sensual (and sexual) awareness, you automatically and inevitably open yourselves up to a deeper spiritual connection. As Charles and Caroline Muir say in their enchanting book, *Tantra: The Art of Conscious Loving,* "Many of us aspire to spiritual growth. But we also desire to grow with a partner. Tantric yoga was the path couples chose thousands of years ago to satisfy this dilemma, since the Tantric discipline allows men and woman to have a mate, to enjoy sex, and to experience spiritual fulfillment, often simultaneously." Among the common techniques that couples use to get into a "Tantric state of mind" is to regularly practice meditation, harmonic breathing (in which they learn to breath in synchronicity), as well as other techniques that awaken, purify, and activate the seven chakras of the body. (If you are interested in learning about Tantric yoga and the energy chakras, please consult the bibliography for further reading.) Here, I've selected four techniques as described by Charles and Caroline Muir that I believe can give a couple—either beginners, intermediates, or advanced students—a very special experience.

- **Contacting Three Points of Pleasure.** This technique is part of a ritual called "nyasa," an advanced form of Tantric touch that charges and awakens the chakras. The woman is in the female-superior position, kneeling above her lover with her chest close to his. The man is deeply inside of her, trying to establish contact with her G spot (AKA sacred spot) with his penis. At the same time, with his index and middle fingers on either side of his penis, the man then places gentle pressure on the woman's anus with his index finger, which adds continued pressure on the woman's G spot, from his penis's opposite direction. Meanwhile, the man presses his middle finger lightly against the woman's clitoris. Being careful not to move, the man then alternates pressure on the three points of pleasure—the G spot, the anus, and the clitoris.

- **Uniting the Energy Poles.** In this technique, the man places gentle pressure from inside on his lover's G spot with his index and middle fingers, while simultaneously his thumb gently stimulates her clitoris. For increased sensation, he can rest his other hand on the mons of her pubic bone, thereby pressuring her G spot from the outside. Again, movement should be kept to a minimum.

- **Kneeling at the Gate of Pleasure.** This technique begins in a male-superior position, with the man inside of his lover; however, he is penetrating her before he is firmly erect. Once the couple is comfortable in this position, the man then lifts the woman's legs onto his shoulders (without withdrawing), and shifts into a kneeling position. From here, he inserts one or two fingers inside of his lover's vagina to gently massage her G spot. His fingers not only stimulate her sacred spot, but also his own penis, which is still inside of her.

- **Heart to Heart Loving.** This technique is performed in Yab Yum position, a position unique to Tantra [**Illustration 39.**] With the lingam (penis) deep inside the yoni (vagina), the nipples of both partners touch. The man begins by breathing out, conscious of his breath and energy moving upward, while at the same he focuses on his penis extending energetically deeper inside of his lover. The woman breathes in her lover's breath, becoming conscious of receiving his energy and pulling it upward through her body into her heart. She then exhales, and the man breathes in her heart energy, bringing it down through his heart to his penis. There is a great visualization component here, with both lovers seeing with their mind's eyes the exchange of energy between them, as it moves between them—heart to heart. Indeed, the Yab Yum position in essence allows for this deep spiritual connection of two hearts, uniting them as one.

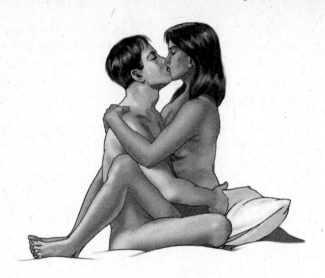

Ill. 39

---

284. *The Deer Exercise for Men.*

This tip highlights the many benefits of extending male sexual arousal and holding back ejaculation. According to Charles and Caroline Muir, when a man learns how to control ejaculation, "He is able to make love for extended periods of time—in fact for as long as he chooses." This increases not only his pleasure, but his lover's pleasure as well—for by arousing her more slowly, he increases her ability to orgasm as well as the intensity of her orgasm once she releases. But men also benefit: the longer a man engages in lovemaking, the more he decreases his refractory period (the time lapse between erections). As the Muirs say, "Since he hasn't spent his sexual energy, he's able to make love again if he wants to, or if his beloved does."

Another expert in the field of sexology, Dr. Stephen Chang, author of the very interesting *The Tao of Sexology*, suggests that men practice The Deer Exercise in order to learn how to extend their arousal cycle and control their ejaculation. The exercise can be done standing, sitting, or lying down, and is performed in two stages, and is best done without clothing. Here is what Dr. Chang suggests:

First stage. The first stage is meant to encourage semen production.

1. Rub the palms of your hands together vigorously to create heat.

2. With your right hand, cup your testicles so that the palm of your hand completely covers them. Without squeezing, allow the heat of your hand to gently pressure the testicles.

3. Place the palm of your left hand on the area of your pubis, once inch below your navel.

4. With a slight pressure so that a gentle warmth begins to build in your pubic area, move your left hand in a clockwise or counterclockwise circle eighty-one times.

5. Rub your hands together again in a vigorous motion.

6. Now reverse the position of your hands, so that your left hand cups your testicles and your right hand is on your pubis. Repeat circular rubbing in the opposite direction another eighty-one times.

As you complete each eighty-one-set cycle, make sure that you concentrate on what you are doing and feel the warmth grow. Concentration is necessary to enhance the results.

Second Stage—This stage tones and strengthens the man's PC (pubococcygeus) muscle.

1. Tighten muscles around your anus and draw them up and in. When done properly, it will feel as if air is being drawn up your rectum. Tighten as hard as you can and hold as long as you can.

2. Stop and relax a moment.

3. Repeat the anal contractions. Do this as many times as you can without feeling discomfort.

In this second stage, focus on a tingling sensation ascending upward from the anus into your lower back. Both exercises can be done daily, weekly, or monthly, and Dr. Chang assures men that they will see immediate results.

285. The Washcloth Trick.

Here is another exercise to strengthen and enhance a man's PC muscle and his sexual responsiveness, and is done most easily in the shower, but you can really do it anywhere you wish. Lay a washcloth across your erect penis. Start by using a dry washcloth as a form of resistance and then graduate to a wet one. Try making your penis jump up and down. If your penis does not actually move, try to do so isometrically. As you become more comfortable, try to practice making the penis jump when erect and do so 2–3 times a day for 2–3 minutes at a time. Behind the Washcloth Trick is further scientific evidence of a direct correlation between orgasmic intensity and a well-toned PC muscle, which of course makes sense since orgasmic pulsations are muscular contractions.

286. Male Multiple Orgasms.

Male multiple orgasm occurs when a man experiences more than one orgasm with the *same* erection. In other words, after an orgasm, he does not lose his erection or go through what is referred to technically as the refractory phase. Instead, he remains erect *and* he has not ejaculated. Most people assume that a man's orgasm and ejaculation are one and the same event, occurring at the moment of peak sexual excitement. Now, I would never dare to argue that two events experienced as one is nothing less than a divine experience; however, for men who experience multiple orgasms, they are aware of the separation of these two events.

So why would on a man want to become multi-orgasmic? Sexual parlour tricks aside, those who have experienced it say their orgasms become longer lasting and more intense and enable a man to prolong lovemaking. As Karl shared, "In two months I went from skeptical to being multiply orgasmic and the self-confidence it gave me has been incredible." For most men, the ejaculation process is about two seconds and this allows a man to extend that process and the sensations involved. The key to a man becoming multi-orgasmic is a well-toned PC muscle and understanding your own ejaculation process, including the timing. Be clear that there are two parts to the ejaculation process: emission (the gun gets loaded) and expulsion (the gun gets fired). When a man is able to control the expulsion phase, because of his awareness of his physiological response and a well-toned PC muscle, he can voluntarily delay or prevent ejaculation. A man will still experience the full sensation of orgasm—complete with rapid heart rate, muscle contractions, and the intense sensation of release. Some men refer to this as a dry orgasm. Any practice of withholding of ejaculation, delaying orgasm, conserving chi, (AKA the life force), all get lumped into this same area. What distinguishes them is the philosophy behind them. For Tantric sex the delay is about the journey of sharing physically and spiritually while blending the energy of partners. For Taoists, delaying orgasm has the practical consequence of deepening the sexual experience. For men who wish to explore these avenues further, there are two terrific books available, Mantak Chia's *The Multi-Orgasmic Male* and Dr. Barbara Keesling's, *How to Make Love All Night*. Both of these books have clear, step-by-step programs, with Chia using line-drawn illustrations.

287. Female Multiple Orgasms.

In comparison, a female multiple orgasm is defined as more than one orgasm in the same lovemaking session. So why do women get off with a broader scope of definition so to speak? The answer is physiological. Blood and oxygen power orgasms, and for women, the increased blood in the pelvis as a result of the sexual stimulation, the vasocongestion of the sexual organs, does not flow out of their sexual organs at the moment of orgasm in the way it does for men who ejaculate. According to Joel Black and Susan Crain Bakos's book, *Sex over 50*, women experience three types of multiple orgasms:

- Compound singles, in which each orgasm is distinct and separated by a partial return to an unaroused state

- Sequential multiples, in which orgasms occur two to ten minutes apart with a minimal reduction in arousal between them

- Serial multiples, in which a woman experiences numerous orgasms separated by mere seconds or minutes, with no diminishment of arousal. Some women say this feels like one long orgasm with spasms of varying intensity

288. Kegels, Kegels, and More Kegels.

This exercise is a standard but powerful exercise for women to increase their sexual sensitivity. By now, we have all heard about Kegels, and most of us know that as long as you have good muscle control, no problems from episiotomies, or other psychological issues, there is no surer way to strengthen the muscles of the pelvic floor than by doing this simple exercise. And remember, as I told the men in the tip above, there is a direct correlation between a toned PC muscle and the intensity of your orgasms. A woman can check her own muscle tone by inserting her fingers into her vagina and then tightening around her fingers. If the muscles surrounding your fingers feel like a thin line, chances are you have some PC muscle work to do. If the muscles create the sensation of a broad, 1/2-inch band, then you are probably in good shape. By doing more Kegels, however, you can go from good to great. The easiest way for you to identify the PC muscle group is by squeezing those muscles that stop the flow of urine. When you stop your flow during urination, you are actually contracting the PC muscle floor and improving their tone. You might be surprised how strong these muscles become once they get going. As with doing any muscle work, vary the degree of contraction, starting with short, intense contractions, holding for ten seconds, and then relaxing for ten seconds. Then tighten again for five seconds, and repeat the cycle until your muscles feel fatigued. Bryce Britton, MS, author of *The Love Muscle*, suggests that after five weeks of doing these Kegel exercises three times daily for five minutes, the woman's PC muscle will become noticeably more toned, and the man will sense her increased tightness.

289. The Instruments.

Aside from straight Kegel exercises, you can take the intensity up a notch by adding weight resistance. The Vaginal Weight Lifting Egg and The Kegelcisor both act in the same way. They give a woman resistance to contracting the PC muscle and increase its workload and speed in toning. Both of the items mentioned above work the same way. First, they give your PC muscle something concrete to squeeze; and second, by adding the weight, you increase the resistance, so your muscle actually works harder. Similar to the way isometric exercises work, the Vaginal Egg is inserted like a tampon; it too has a string that allows for easy removal. And like a tampon, the Egg allows a woman to walk around and do light work while wearing it, providing heightened awareness of the PC muscle working to keep it in. Additionally, the woman can add weight to the egg's string to increase the speed of results. Some women have done tip 291 (Hip

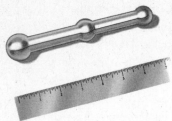

Rolls) while wearing their eggs. The Kegelcisor is inserted halfway and is used while lying down. Best to watch in a mirror and get personal feedback on your contractions.

290. Great Lover Moment: Ladies, Suck Him into You.

This tip came from a woman, let's call her Christine, who shared in a seminar how to give a man the sensation of being sucked into you. During intercourse, just as the head of his glans is about to enter the woman, she breathes out as much as she can; and then, milliseconds later, just as the head has started to enter her, she breathes in very deeply while at the same time strongly contracting her PC muscle. When Christine first did this, her boyfriend exclaimed, "What did you just do? It feels like you just sucked me into you." Quite a neat trick, wouldn't you say, ladies?

291. Hip Roll, Here We Come.

For those of you who have a dance background, hip rolls are a great way to tighten the entire pelvic floor. One mother of four, and a recent grandmother, who has been an erotic dancer for twenty years said her boyfriends have all said she is the tightest woman with whom they have ever been. She totally attributes her incredibly toned PC muscles to the constant hip rolls of her dancing career. For those of you without a dance background, here is how they're done:

1. Stand with your feet hip-width apart.

2. Imagine there is a dotted line down the center of your body, from the crown of your head through the floor.

3. Imagine that the line extending down the center of your body has a pencil point on the end; your job is to make the point of that pencil draw circles with your motions.

4. Next, imagine that there is a dotted line circling your hips about two inches from your body. You are going to move your hips within that circle.

5. Now begin to roll your hips or move them in a circular motion, first in one direction, and then in the other. Try not to bend your knees, and instead let the motion come from your pelvic region.

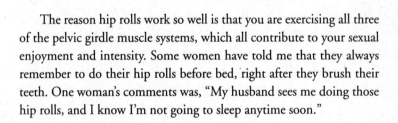

The reason hip rolls work so well is that you are exercising all three of the pelvic girdle muscle systems, which all contribute to your sexual enjoyment and intensity. Some women have told me that they always remember to do their hip rolls before bed, right after they brush their teeth. One woman's comments was, "My husband sees me doing those hip rolls, and I know I'm not going to sleep anytime soon."

How to Be a Great Lover in Fantasy

$\mathcal{T}$his section was inspired by a recent trend I have been observing in my sexuality seminars: that more and more women and men are interested in, paying attention to, and honoring their sexual fantasies. Unlike what is often represented in the male entertainment industry, fantasies don't have to be salacious or gratuitous. The fact of the matter is, a fantasy, by definition, is a sexual feeling captured by a particular scenario, image, or action. It's the feeling that people are after; the scenario is often simply the outfit on the mannequin, as it were. In this section, I have gathered a smorgasbord of delights that may just trigger your fancy, or that of your lover, or in some cases, the both of you. As you peruse and perhaps play, remember that these suggestions are additions, not staples, to your sexual feast. They are not about replacing your partner, they are about enhancing and expanding what you and your partner have. Great Lovers know that fantasies are just that—*not* real.

292. Give Yourself and Your Partner Permission to Discuss Any Fantasy.

Remember the tip about creating an environment of emotional safety? Well, this tip is directly related to that one. In fact, before you and your partner can go near acting out your fantasies—either his or hers—you absolutely must feel safe and secure in your relationship, which means that you must feel comfortable enough to voice whatever it is you so desire. But before you get to the point of voicing that secret fantasy, you need to be able to extend full permission—to both of you. So here's a checklist to see if you've truly given full permission:

- Have you already determined what turns you both on and off?

- Have you established an environment of emotional safety, in which you both trust each other with your most vulnerable feelings?

- Are you comfortable with how each of you likes to be aroused?

- Are you willing to accept whatever it is your partner wants in terms of a sexual fantasy, and accept it in a nonjudgmental way?

- Are you ready to be honest and say when you are comfortable or not comfortable?

If you can answer these questions in the affirmative, then you are more than likely ready and willing to grant permission to explore your fantasies.

293. Ask Your Partner for a Fantasy You Haven't Been Able to Voice in the Past.

One couple I worked with told me their own story: Together for six years, Tom had always been afraid to tell Marty about his favorite sexual fantasy. It was only after they began to explore each other in other ways (experimenting with toys, having sex blindfolded) that Tom ventured forth. He told Marty that his ultimate fantasy was to watch an erotic film of two women with her. The turn-on for Tom was watching Marty's reaction to the film. Although Marty had never thought of being with another woman, she was completely game to watch the film with Tom, whom she trusted completely. As soon as they sat down in front of their DVD screen, their excitement began to mount—both because of what was happening on-screen (a tasteful seduction scene set in a mountainside cabin by California's Big Sur), and by what was happening with each other. Marty loved watching Tom get so turned on, and became more and more aroused herself. Soon, they had forgotten about the video altogether and were all over each other like honeymooners.

Tom and Marty's fantasy is just one example of how voicing a fantasy can unleash tremendous passion and fresh energy into your sex life. Marty and Tom had no complaints about their sexual relationship; in fact, they were highly satisfied with it. But when they discovered how intoxicating sharing their fantasies could be, there was no turning back.

294. Get in Touch with the Feeling Fueling Your Fantasy.

Do you want to be seduced? Do you want to be dominated? Is your hottest dream to be "taught" by your man or woman? Maybe you want to be that seductress no man can resist? Perhaps the stern master with the firm hand is your dream come true? As soon as the feeling behind the fantasy is crystallized, then you have a whole range of scenarios available to satisfy that appetite. The firm hand could be that of the teacher to the student, the queen to her subject, or perhaps delivered by the slavemaster to an unruly slave. Once you know the feelings and emotions you wish to evoke, acting out a fantasy is a bit like choosing the type of TV program you prefer: As with DirecTV, you select from a range of options.

295. Give Yourself Permission to Get into Character.

Whether it is a change of speech, posture, or apparel, the strength of fantasies is in one's ability to assume that role, to get into that character much like an actor does. The easiest way to explain why this works is to get in touch with how you regularly become a different persona or feel differently when you are wearing formal evening wear or your workout clothes. Both outfits (and their accompanying personas) serve a purpose and change how you feel about yourself. Getting into the character in a fantasy is no different. In that way, your sexual fantasy and character transition is greatly enhanced by introducing different articles of dress or behavior, be it the British accent of the lord of the manor, or full dominatrix leather garb complete with whip and mask. And if appropriate, give yourself the freedom to enhance with sexual props.

296. Try the Domination/Submission Fantasy.

This is one of the easiest fantasy roles for couples to introduce. Why? Because the power dynamic is so clearly spelled out and it can be done just about anywhere. Every group of animals, and let's be honest, that's what we humans are at our core, has a power hierarchy that determines who gets to do what first or to whom, so these lovers are accessing one of Mother Nature's better gifts to sexual behavior—the hierarchy of power. Perhaps the woman wears only a choker, stilettos, and a full length cape over her completely nude body in public because her sexual master wants her to be constantly available for him. Or the woman ties her man to the stair railing with his tie, and then proceeds to arouse him mercilessly so his penis will be exactly as she pleases. Whatever the scenario, the couple knows the incredible sexual heat of mastering this power reciprocity.

297. Try the Voyeuristic/Exhibitionistic Fantasy.

Seeing and being seen are two basic human drives that center around attention, and simply put, human beings thrive with attention and wither without it. Attention is one part of this tip; the other is knowing you are making your partner hot just by letting them watch. Brain sex is how one woman describes this type of fantasy play. "When our house was being remodeled, my husband had a small interior room with a viewing window cut into the upper wall of our master bathroom because he loves to watch me when I am bathing. And I love to change positions and 'views' for him and knowing that as I am doing myself with the showerhead on the edge of our giant Jacuzzi tub, he is going totally out of his mind and jerking off in his own little room."

298. Ménage à Trois.

This fantasy, especially two women with one man, has become more common due to its incredibly standard presentation in porn films. Alas, more proof that we are very programmable: What we see, we tend to want. For men, this fantasy resonates with their desire to be able to satisfy two women at one time, the manly man thing. The thinking goes as follows: The two women will be into each other until a "real" man comes along and takes care of "business" properly. For a woman, being with their male lover and another woman is usually a form of sexual exploration and expansion of how she sees herself sexually. Two caveats: First, women often feel pressured into trying this fantasy for a male partner; but instead of it opening up their sexual horizons, it closes them down because she feels pressured or manipulated. And secondly, the two women can often find each other so interesting they might leave the man on the sidelines, not likely his preferred position.

Of course there are ménage à trois arrangements among two men and one woman, but these seem less common—more than likely because two men is too many, inspiring male competition. But, as in life in general, such threesomes do exist, and one woman who has explored this territory, reported, "It was fantastic—it was like having two male love slaves—I was totally into it!"

299. Swinging.

Like the ménage à trois, swinging involves multiple partners. And recently, I have heard reports of an increase in requests for this sexual fantasy, and, for some, this lifestyle. Swinging is defined as couples who switch partners. However, what begins usually with a man's desire to be with other women can backfire. Swinging protocol typically includes that all parties involved be in couples (so as to lessen the likelihood of predatory single males trying to join in) and that the woman does the approaching. And though some couples happily enjoy swinging, and sharing each other with other like-minded couples, some couples find it more difficult to avoid the fallout. As it was explained to me, swinging can result in some women experiencing a sexual epiphany, becoming more sexually aware and empowered—always a good thing. But if she splits off from her mate, then what started out as his fantasy quickly turns into his nightmare: She ends up leaving him in the dust. The emotional impact of this fantasy can be an unbelievable experience of sharing, but it can also yield a convoluted emotional net. Of all the fantasies, this is the one for which you need to be most clear about your intentions.

300. Indulge His Dress-Up Fantasy.

Playing with gender roles can be a potent form of fantasy seduction. What are the roles some people like to assume? Some men, for instance, like to dress up as the other sex. One couple—he is a competitive triathlete and she is a landscape architect—shared this provocative fantasy with me in a sexuality seminar: George liked for his wife, Candace, to buy women's lingerie—for him to wear. The moment of the fantasy began when George visualized his wife picking out and purchasing the lingerie—just for him. That she accepts and wants to do this for him is probably the hottest part of this for him. Once he'd received the "package," he'd quietly get dressed in the bathroom and then ask her to meet him in the bedroom. As Candace explained, "The whole thing takes on an edgy feeling—as a couple, George's fantasy brings us closer because it's so private, so personal." When I asked her if she was at all uncomfortable about George's desire to dress in women's lingerie, she said adamantly, "No. Not at all! This is just a feature of his sexual personality—I know how hot I make him in bed. I don't worry. I'm just glad he finally shared this with me. And I get really excited, too."

301. The Bored Housewife and Cabana Boy.

Many a sexually emancipated woman has dreamed of hiring her own private gigolo. Do any of you remember the sparks that flew when Richard Gere hit the screen in *American Gigolo*? Or why *The Graduate* felt so edgy? Why Geena Davis's character succumbs to Brat Pitt's bad boy in *Thelma and Louise*? These films capture the essence of why this fantasy works for some women: The woman is either older or more economically powerful, but she is at the mercy of her desire for the young stud. This situation allows for a certain lack of attachment between the "cabana boy" and the "wife" that, in turn, can allow for more uninhibited sex. And this fantasy appeals to some men as well—men who enjoy being at the mercy of a sexually driven and powerful woman. Try it on for size.

302. The Prostitute and the Gentleman.

There is a reason men have sought out paid sex workers for centuries—because they like the simplicity of the money-for-sex arrangement. For the sake of a fantasized event, if the power situation of this sort appeals to you, you and your lover might find it fun. If for the moment, both of you are playing out this scenario, then you are restricting your personal (or emotional) involvement while wearing the so-called costumes of working girl and customer, and when the role of those personalities is in place, then you have more freedom to explore the sexual situation itself. One couple who came to a sexuality seminar shared an experience they had in which they checked into a hotel for an overnight stay. Having packed their bags with appropriate clothing, they pretended: he was a customer; she was an expensive call girl. They ordered champagne; they lit the gas fireplace; they let go of their "regular selves" and assumed their new identities. The hilarious part happened when they were checking out and the valet, while waiting for his tip, accidentally spilled their treasure chest of sexual goodies in the Ritz-Carlton driveway.

303. The Officer and the Gentlewoman.

This fantasy scenario was shared in one of my sexuality seminars by a man who otherwise was a gentle, laid-back executive. He related that he and his fiancée had explored many fantasy scenarios, but he never felt that he could ask for his number-one fantasy: wanting to say "Suck me, bitch!" and demand she suck him while he dominated the encounter. His fear was that she would be turned off and find his request disrespectful, which means that he would then be cut off from sex. As with all things in life, we never really know what someone else is thinking, and when she said, "I have no problem with that, it might actually be fun." He almost went out of his mind planning his fantasy's perfect execution.

It unfolded as follows when they went away two weeks later. In one of his small carry-on bags were carefully chosen items, specifically two costumes—one for him and one for her. His was a naval officer's dress uniform; hers was a neat, slightly old-fashioned long, black, silk dress with a white, lace collar. His fantasy was for her to "take him orally" in front of a mirror while she was on her knees, the front of her dress unbuttoned and showcasing her Aubade lace bra (he had purchased it especially for the event), the back of the dress lifted to expose her bare derriere while he stood over her and leaned against the wall, watching it all in the mirror. Now, obviously the two of them had to completely trust each other; otherwise, the power play of such a situation might feel uncomfortable, even intimidating. But this couple did share utmost trust in themselves, their relationship, and each other, so exploring this fantasy became a way to explore their erotic personas. All they need to do to trigger a replay is place his officer's cap on their dresser.

304. Phone Sex.

Now, this may be a fantasy for some and a regular routine for others. Either way, having phone sex can be a lusty, playful way to break up your sexual routine—especially if one or both of you ever travels. What usually unfolds is that the two of you are connected via the telephone, and one or both of you makes a suggestive remark, such as, "What are you wearing?" Or get right to the point by saying, "I am touching myself right now—do you want to know where?" Of course, your partner is sharing with you what he or she is doing on the other end, as you describe what you are doing on your end. Sex-by-wire can be hot, hot, hot. Some couples have started fantasy scenarios via phone sex and then taken them to intense levels when they get together. Phone sex is also a great time to experiment with self-pleasuring methods and new novelties.

305. "Daddy, I've Been Bad."

This fantasy plays into the bad little girl who needs "discipline" from her so-called daddy. For many couples, the agreed-upon discipline is a spanking, which gets some women very turned on. But invariably the heat for the man comes from the woman saying, "I've been bad." Ladies, don't worry that you might feel silly saying this; chances are, at first you will feel a bit silly. But what most women have shared with me is that the reaction this line creates for him is so amazing, it doesn't take long for them to get used to how instantly this line hits his switch and how suddenly you know a few simple words that can rock his world. Sometimes this fantasy play culminates in a rear-entry doggie position with the man administering gentle to very firm slaps on her bottom, letting her be the guide of intensity by asking, "How bad have you been?" But do not think this is about inflicting pain; it isn't. You can modify the scenario by having the woman turn up the heat by whispering to her man that she has been a bad girl at work and he has to discipline her. The result invariably is more intense sex.

306. Innocent Schoolgirl.

The flirty, pleated, tartan skirt with the starched, oxford cloth shirt pulled tautly over pert breasts is the source of many fantasies for both sexes. The power of this fantasy is rooted in the power of burgeoning and ripening sexuality as evidenced by a sexually blossoming teenage girl. Some consider meting out detentions and appropriate discipline because her knee socks are falling down. Or she had a mark on her blouse, of course in a strategic location. From sitting on her boyfriend's lap and enjoying his caresses to a rosy spanked derriere of a truant schoolgirl over the knee of her headmaster to being the perfect lab specimen, this fantasy scenario can expand in many different directions.

307. Nurse Nancy and Doctor Dan.

This is the grown-up version of "playing doctor." As with the schoolgirl scenario, there are many different ways to play this fantasy out. Either partner can be an examining doctor, nurse, or patient. There is a vulnerability created by open paper robes or a mere sheet covering your totally nude body. And for some, the use of medical props greatly expands the sensations they can create. The coolness of the stethoscope on an erect nipple, a speculum to complete an internal exam—these are just two stimulating tips. Perhaps the female doctor needs to see how long he can last during intense oral stimulation. And when in character, any medical treatment or swallowing of your medicine can take on new meanings. Part dominance, part submission—the choice is that of the parties involved.

308. True Lies.

Re-create the scene in *True Lies* in which Jamie Lee Curtis strips for Schwarzenegger. Let me set the stage for you: Secret agent Harry Tasker (Arnold Schwarzenegger) is enmeshed in trying to stop a gang of international terrorists from getting their hands on missing nuclear weapons, while Helen (Jamie Lee Curtis), feeling neglected, begins a covert affair with a sleazy used-car salesman pretending to be a spy. When Harry finds out, he decides to give Helen a lesson in spy games, which backfires when the couple is kidnapped and stuck in the middle of an international terrorist crisis. The best part of this scene is the moment the omniscient audience becomes aware that she is stripping for her husband in order to save him. Many couples play this video and then go on to re-create their own scene. If you want some private tutoring beforehand, consider getting the best instructional video I've seen, "The Art of Exotic Dancing for Everyday Women," instruction by Laurie Conrad. This video, available at www.phillyfilms.com, is a great way to learn some amazing erotic dance moves.

309. From Here to Eternity.

Re-create the beach scene with Deborah Kerr and Burt Lancaster in the 1953 film *From Here to Eternity*. Overcome with illicit desire, the two of them fall into each other's arms at the water's edge—semiclothed, kissing in full throttle. Hot, moist, skin on skin, surges of motion from the waves and they are so into each other they can't be broken apart. This scene captures the kind of sexual intensity and focus we all should experience. It is no wonder many couples find the thought of sex on a beach, in a pool, or body of water very tantalizing. Be aware, however, that water is definitely not a lubricating solution. To the contrary, it will wash away what Mother Nature provides. So if you attempt to re-create this scene, you may need to bring your own lubrication, otherwise it can make for reduced motion. And, as many beach lovers have shared, be careful about sand in your bathing suit and other delicate areas.

310. Bull Durham.

Re-create the scene in *Bull Durham* when Kevin Costner swipes the table clean and thrusts Susan Sarandon down on top. The arm sweep of "get it out of the way" in this scene actually represents the degree of focus we want our partner to have on us during sex. The resulting sexual explosion that then takes place on the table spells, "I can't wait and nothing is going to stop me!" This kind of momentum gets you so hot for your partner that neither can stop the buildup, so you use whatever available surface is nearby—table, tub, or wall. Gentlemen, this is a major female fantasy (minus breaking all the dishes—even if you are Greek—and having to clean up the mess)!

311. Talk Dirty.

The first part of this fantasy is to find out which terms do and do not work for you, and it's best to do so outside the bedroom. As some couples have shared, it is an absolutely hilarious thing to talk about over lattes on Sunday at a coffee house. The reason talking dirty is a fantasy is that partners tend to lose themselves in the passion. Because you are being so much more explicit in your sexual demands, you also tend to become more animalistic in your behavior, making for very hot sex. For people who cherish this fantasy, the turn-on comes from the-coarser-the-better language. Note to self, my gentlemen readers: Let the woman set the pace for the level of explicitness. Let her take the lead: She may start with saying she likes your penis, then wants your dick, and then wants you to fuck her with your cock. This way you can match her level and not go too far and upset the mood. Also, realize that not everyone responds to talking dirty. All the more reason to talk about it beforehand and start out mild, only escalating after gauging your partner's interest. I've had women tell me it was all they could do to not burst out laughing when a lover started using explicit language, and some men who were caught off guard by their ladies' vocalizations in the heat of the moment. But here's a classic in-the-moment example that worked and worked beautifully. It comes from a female executive who found out quite innocently how to stoke her man's fires with her spicy language. They had started to indulge in activity while standing on her balcony; he had lifted her dress and had entered her from behind. She was matching his thrusts when she turned her head and whispered to him, "I want you to f__k me." At first he couldn't believe his ears: This was his all-time fantasy and she had done it without his having to ask. He was trying to maintain a steady motion and the dam broke when she turned again and said, "I believe I told you to f__k me." So perhaps your English professor was right: Never underestimate the power of language.

312. How to Create Your Own Fantasies.

I have created a way for my readers and viewers to create their own fantasies. It is a game I call "Finish the Fantasy." You start with a sentence and then together use your own creative juice to complete the storyline, creating your own fantasy. Favorite starter sentences include:

"She is walking away from me wearing a red, silk robe when she drops it and ____."

"He walks in the door and he has ____ in his hand."

"The phone rang and ____."

"He asked her to meet him ____."

"She passed by him every day on the subway ___."

"No one told her the new professor would be so ____."

"She just loved a man in uniform ____."

Fill in the blanks with whatever erotic ideas come to mind. Some couples will even take things a bit further by alternating sentences so that they both have input in the fantasy's direction.

313. *Incorporate Toys to Expand Your Lovemaking Options.*

Just as you have learned to grant each other permission to explore your fantasies in general, it's also important to grant that same permission to experiment with toys. Toys are fun. Toys do not replace either one of you. They quite simply and wonderfully enhance the fun factor of your sexual experience. Below are ten tips that give you all the most current information on how to use toys and what toys to use. You can find these products at many places; consult the resource list at the back of the book for more information.

314. *Lubricants for You and Your Toys.*

These little bottles of fun can so enhance what you are already doing, I am surprised that more people do not know about them. Whether you are using a lubricant for either partner or assisting in prolonging an intercourse session, the main aim of these products is to ease motion in those most delicate areas and enhance sensation. If you use latex condoms for protection, you must use a water-based product, as anything with an oil or petroleum substrate (massage oils, hand lotions, baby oil) are the mortal enemy of latex and start to erode their protection capabilities.

CATEGORIES:

- Water-based, glycerine-free: Slippery Stuff or Femglide (same product, only marketed to medical groups), Liquid Silk, and Maximus.

- Water-based, containing glycerine. These are enjoyed by people who do not have a problem with yeast infections: Very Private, Sensura, and Sex Grease.

- Very Private was recently given the "Seal of Approval" by OBGYN.net for all their products associated with women's health.

- Flavored: Midnite Fire.

One main rule: if anything is going to be inserted into the body, make sure you use a water-based lubricant and be careful about any dyes and flavored products. It is difficult for the vagina to cleanse itself of inserted oils, and residue from any inserted product can upset the natural balance of organisms in the vagina and result in an overgrowth of normal bacteria and/or yeast.

315. Vibrators—External/Internal.

Just about any area of the body has a vibrator designed for it. When considering a product, look at where you might use it: on her clitoris, the sides of her labia, under his scrotum, on his or her nipples, or inserted anally for either of you. Are you using it alone or with a partner? How strong or intense do you want the vibrator to be? How quiet do you want it to be? Do you need it to be water resistant so you can use it in the shower?

Vibrators also come in several basic styles: phallus-shaped and hands-free/remote control. There are also those that are disguised to look like tubes of lipstick or blush brushes. For gentlemen who are worried a vibrator will replace them, fear not. Women constantly state that although vibrators are fast (let's be serious, no man can attain 50,000 oscillations per minute), nothing will ever replace the feel of a man's body. I advise you gentlemen to simply make yourself a part of her pleasure by trying your hand at being in charge of the controls. Here are some specific products you might find interesting:

CLASSICS

- **The Pocket-Rocket**—a small, single-speed style powered by two AA batteries. Many companies make these, varying in colors and names.

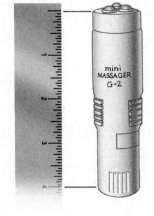

- **Rabbit Pearl**—Almost all toys with the rabbit, bunny, or wabbit name variation is a knock-off of this original design. The Rabbit Pearl has two operative areas: The first is the inserted wand section that rotates the pearl segment for stimulating the sensitive first one and a half inches of the woman's vagina (hence the pearl name); and the second feature is the vibrating molded rabbit, whose long, flexible ears and smooth nose can create incredible sensation on the clitoris.

- ***Hitachi Magic Wand***—this is a large, plug-in electric wand that is best used with the cushioning effect of a washcloth, as it may be too intense to use "bareback."

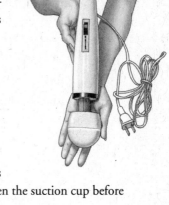

- ***Nipple Vibrators***—these vibrators are specifically molded for nipples. These can be attached with a small adjustable clamp or with air suction. Some people find the vibrators attach better when they moisten the suction cup before applying.

NEW AND IMPROVED

- ***The Tongue Joy***—Perhaps the cutest thing I have seen in a long time, this vibrator is the brainchild of a medical equipment executive who created it after seeing a CNN special on tongue piercing. He realized that the stud was being used for oral stimulation and thought that adding vibration would be a terrific idea. Not wanting to pierce his tongue, his wife gave him the idea for how to attach the gizmo to a nonpierced tongue—the rest is history. The Tongue Joy comes with three different sized, highly stretchable rings with a small pierced hole. The I-shaped vibrator segment can be powered by either small watch batteries or the more intense power of a

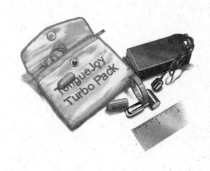

two AA battery pack. Most couples use the smaller battery barbell during oral sex, since the elastic band keeps it in place. The larger ring is designed to be worn at the base of the man's shaft, and the smaller ring can position the vibrator directly on the chosen area or make the fingertip itself a vibrator. All Tongue Joy products include batteries when purchased.

- ***The Femme Line***—from Candida Royalle. These nonphallic-shaped vibrators are more gentle and especially good for sensitive women and those wishing to try vibrators for the first time.

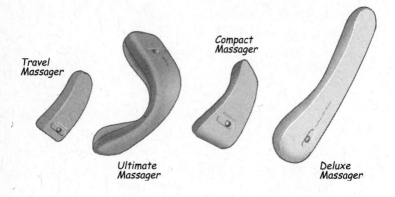

Travel Massager

Compact Massager

Ultimate Massager

Deluxe Massager

- ***Multi-Satisfier***—Microchip processors lend their range of options to vibrators. You have your choice of five speeds, five vibration styles, and with or without a rotating feature. It has a most user-friendly backlit faceplate so you can see what you are doing under the covers.

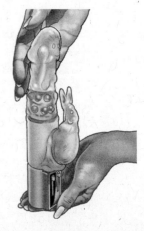

316. *Bondage Light.*

The best all-around set I know of is Sportsheets. Designed by a U.S. Marine whose inspiration came from a David Letterman show in which the comedian was Velcroed to the wall. And should you wish to try more homegrown items to tie each other up with, a scarf or tie can fit the bill.

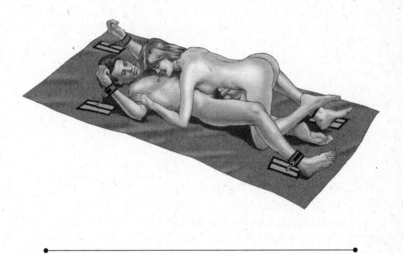

317. *Goodies That Vary the Senses.*

Any textured item can be used on or worn by the individual to vary the sensation of touch, so that your other senses such as sight or hearing can become more concentrated. Whether that item is soft like leather or rougher like fur, you can expand skin play. You can also try anything from flavored dusting powder to chocolate paint and a brush to spice things up. Or pop an Altoid mint and then apply your artist's mouth to your lover's body and see the results.

318. Dildos.

Anything that can be inserted—
whether it vibrates or not, is designed
in the shape of a penis or not, or meant
to resemble a creature or a plant—can
be used as a dildo.

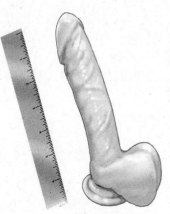

319. PVC Molded Toys.

There are many toys made of this pliable material that can bring wonderful pleasure to both of you, including seminar favorites: the Pink
Elephant, including a new style with adjustable pearls in the shaft that
can be used by the man solo or by the partner on him; Shaft Sleeves;
and of course a variety of cock rings.

The Pink Elephant (**illustration 51**) (my name for it) is a very soft
5" by 2" hyper-stretchy sleeve that envelops a
man's erect penis and can be used to
create sensation of either vaginal or
anal penetration. First step is to add a
warmed water-based lubricant into
the central shaft and encase his erect
penis.

At this point the creation of sensation is limited only by one's imagination
in using a combination of twisting and up-
and-down strokes. There are two styles: one

with small soft ridges internally that mimic the natural rugae inside of a woman's vagina and the other has a softer interior to mimic anal penetration.

SHAFT SLEEVES

These one-and-a-half-inch tubular sleeves are made of a transparent, nontoxic PVC material. The soft, nubby ridges on the surface are what drive men and women wild with a different kind of sensation. Here's how you can use them:

1. **Woman on her partner.** Slip one over one or two fingers and let them help you pleasure him manually.

2. **Man on his partner,** either manually or during intercourse. When you are pleasuring her manually, this added sensation on her clitoris may increase her stimulation. During intercourse, you can pleasure her by wearing a shaft sleeve at the base of your penis.

3. **On a vibrator.** When you slip a sleeve on your favorite wand vibrator, you've just given it a whole new feel.

COCK RINGS

Cock rings work under the principle of fluid hydraulics: When a penis is stimulated, there is an increase in blood flow into the penis chambers. Then gravity and a drop-off of stimulation cause the blood flow to reverse. Cock rings work to temporarily restrict the blood vessels alongside of the erect penis to reduce the drop-off of penile blood pressure. The result is a firmer, longer-lasting erection, as well as a reported delay in ejaculation for some men. As seen in **illustration 53,** they are to be worn both at the base of the shaft and over the scrotum, in order to heighten the buildup of pressure during stimulation. Some couples have the man wear the cock ring during intercourse, and then remove the ring prior to the man climaxing, or putting it on halfway through intercourse and finish with it in place.

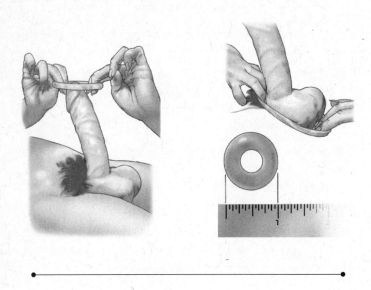

320. *Anal Toys.*

These toys can be used by either partner to enhance the orgasmic sensation by providing a form of resistance for the PC (pubococcygeus) muscle to contract against during orgasm. Such toys include anal beads, which are inserted and worn until the moment of orgasm, when they are either jogged back and forth or pulled out to further stimulate the rhythmically contracting

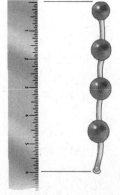

anus. Other toys for this area are the vibrating or nonvibrating butt plugs with the flanged base to prevent its slipping inside. Some men find that the simultaneous stimulation of vibration on the prostate and of the penis can be an off-the-charts sensation.

321. Harnesses.

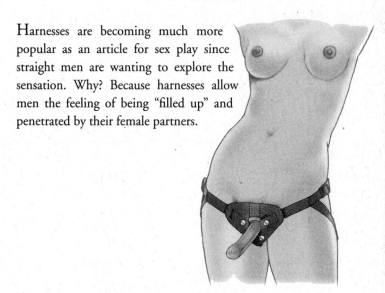

Harnesses are becoming much more popular as an article for sex play since straight men are wanting to explore the sensation. Why? Because harnesses allow men the feeling of being "filled up" and penetrated by their female partners.

322. Great Lover Moment: Video Cameras, Beware.

This tip evolved from one particularly hilarious story that a couple—Jane and Mark—shared with me. True techno-enthusiasts, both Jane and Mark love to play with their equipment, in this case their dildo-cum-video camera, called the Video Voyeur. They have found enormous fun and pleasure from videotaping their sexual escapades with each other. However, Mark was unduly surprised during a recent camping trip with his buddies. When one of his friends asked to borrow Mark's flashlight, the friend opened the box only to find that special video camera that doubles as a dildo. "Oh my God," exclaimed Mark, "That's my wife's dildo!" You can imagine how both Mark and Jane felt about such public airing of their private life: completely embarrassed. Jane had hidden her Video Voyeur in the flashlight box. But there is a more serious warning inherent in this tip: the ease of using our digital and video cameras matches the ease in which the film can be transferred— whether to a flashlight box or . . . the Internet.

323. *The Pearl Necklace.*

Ladies, your man will love what you can do with your pearls. First, lightly lubricate his penis and the pearls, then slowly wrap the pearls around the shaft on one layer, like a choker. Keep hold of the clasp so you don't unintentionally nick him. When his penis is completely encased in your pearls, gently begin to stroke him with an up-and-down rotating motion using the Basket Weave stroke (Tip 240), as indicated

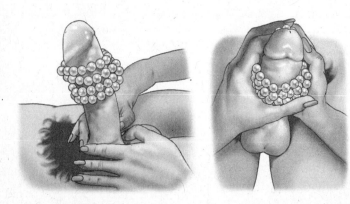

in the illustrations. You can then unfurl the pearls and stroke underneath his testicles, massaging the perineal area. After you're done (or he's done), "coil the poiles" at the base of his shaft and settle yourself on top of him. Never again say diamonds are a girl's best friend—pearls are just as rich a natural resource. And ladies, invest in a set of costume pearls—because you are using lubricant to ease the motion; real pearls do not enjoy getting moisture inside of the pearl (and neither does the silk stranding). A 30–36" strand of 8–10mm round pearls works great.

Frequently Asked Questions and Other New Information on the Sexual Frontier

This section is filled with questions that frequently come up in my sexuality seminars. I figure, if people keep asking the same group of questions, there are plenty of other people out there who want to know the same information. I've also included in this section significant cutting edge or otherwise pertinent information that relates to sexual health that I think you would want to know. By nature, I have an insatiable curiosity for new information and realize after ten years there are many more like me who have the same information appetite.

324. How Do I Know If She's Faking?

First I will explain why women fake it, and then I will guide you on how to tell physiologically if indeed she has faked an orgasm. This is a combination answer, addressing two things about the performance pressure on both sexes. Men are told they have to give a woman an orgasm or they are lovers of questionable ability; at the same time, women get the message that they have to have an orgasm in order to give evidence that he is doing the right things and they are appropriately responsive. Both sides of this message take away from the real purpose of intimacy: our enjoyment. When I have responded to men's questions about how they can learn to tell when a woman is faking, I say this: "If you are going by the standard depictions in the media, chances are you won't be able to tell." Here is why. The depictions of female orgasmic response in the porn industry, men's magazines, and bodice-ripping novels that have a woman swoon upon penetration and/or orgasm are woefully inaccurate. This programming would have us all believe that women yell like banshees, claw backs like animals, and lose consciousness—all thanks to their partner's sexual prowess, his large member, his position either on top or from behind, thrusting like mad. And of course they orgasm together. Now that is not to say all of the above cannot happen in the heat and passion of sex, but these are not standard and shouldn't be expected as inevitable. Sure, some women and men do experience orgasms this way; but definitely not all women and not all the time. That is like saying your sexual response has to be exactly like someone else's. How absurd. Many women and men are very quiet and totally into the pleasure; while others tend to lose themselves in their body's responses and make their distinctively personal sounds or exclamations. (Note: I said distinctively personal.)

But back to the subject at hand. A woman fakes it for two main reasons: 1) she does not want her partner to feel he is not doing a good job; and/or 2) she assumes or knows that she is not going to orgasm, so she fakes it to give a sense of completion to the sexual encounter. Why do women jump to this conclusion so easily? There are a few possibilities: 1) She may be prone to soreness or dryness; 2) They are doing something that isn't working for her or she doesn't like; 3) Or perhaps she is at a certain point of her cycle when she is less sexually sensitive. Many women report "just wanting to get it over with"—either in her own frustration, or in anger at her partner. But let me make this final statement: Men fake it too, and sometimes for the exact same reasons. For the record, gentlemen, here is how you tell if she has orgasmed: Pay attention to the first inch of the vaginal entry, which is where the involuntary (read: not under control) PC (pubococcygeus) muscle contractions occur as part of the orgasmic response. No woman can mimic the speed (0.8 of a second) and intensity of the contraction of the PC muscle during orgasm. She may be able to mimic the sounds, the breathing, the hip writhing, but not these little telltale contractions. As one man described it, "some women just seem to clamp down."

325. How Do I Tell My Lover That I've Been Faking?

Very carefully. In this scenario, I would always suggest you err on the side of diplomacy rather than the harshness of broad daylight facts. With diplomacy as your guide, I would recommend taking what is already happening and expand on it, in the way that will create the sensations and pleasure you want or want to try. This is a much better tactic than telling your partner when he is in the middle of doing his best to please you. I will share with you that I know of a number of relationships that withered after a woman told a man she had been faking all along. If you remember, even Seinfeld, Mr. Sensitive himself, was mortified to find out Elaine had faked. So how do you get him to change what he is doing so you can have an orgasm without having to tell him you've been faking all along? Suggestions from women who have walked successfully through this minefield include: 1) Be clear on what he does that works and ask him to repeat your "favorite"; 2) If you've never actually experienced an orgasm with him, then try to build on what brought you the closest to the point of orgasm, or what felt the most pleasurable; 3) You can guide him by asking him if he is doing something different from the last time you were together. Let him know that you seemed to be feeling more or different sensations. Was he using a slightly different angle? Smoother fingertips? However you decide to address this issue, walk in his moccasins and think about how you would want to be told if he was the one who had been faking. You may decide you would not want to be told at all; and finally, 4) Stop Faking!!!!!! Men are the most amazing downloading devices. If you give them information/reactions that they think works, they will use this information again and again. So if you began by giving him inaccurate information, correct yourself and stop the cycle of sexual deceit. And if your relationship ends, he will take your bad information into his next relationship and no doubt tell the next woman, "Well, it worked for my old girlfriend."

326. How Can I Have an Orgasm with Intercourse?

Let me begin by telling you that most women ask this question because they feel they should be able to orgasm during man-on-top intercourse. This pressure often comes from their partners and the culturing we have about sexual performance. Please be aware that most women orgasm from oral and manual stimulation (with or without a partner), and the reason is very simple. These forms of stimulation stay in constant and close, small-motion contact with the most sensitive areas of a woman's genitals, especially her clitoris. Male-superior (man on top) intercourse often has the man breaking such contact due to his in-and-out pelvic thrusting.

But those women who do orgasm during penetrative intercourse often do so as a result of *already* being highly stimulated. During intercourse, they either get on top and are in charge of the motions and sensations, thereby controlling their own sensations and degrees of stimulation, or they have already reached orgasm from manual or oral stimulation or with a vibrator, and take this stimulation with them into intercourse. When a woman orgasms, she experiences a blood-rush to her pelvic region, and since orgasms are powered by blood and oxygen, this vasocongestion makes it easier for her to climax again during intercourse.

327. I'm Embarrassed to Tell My Husband I Fantasize During Sex. Is There Anything Wrong with That?

Okay, let's start with removing the embarrassment factor. Know that you are in good company, as the majority of people fantasize in some manner or form and the "why" people fantasize is likely to make you feel even more comfortable exploring yours. Quite simply, they are using their brains and imaginations to kick-start, enhance, and add variety to their intimate experiences while remaining committed and monogamous. Think about it: in our day-to-day lives, we have constant role shifts and daydreaming/fantasizing occurs regularly. You are a wife, a mother, a daughter, and an accountant. All of these require you to assume different behaviors, and chances are you daydream about something you'd like to have, that vacation trip, that house, that car, be a size X. Have legs like hers, etc. So if you have these kinds of mental wanderings in daily public life, why wouldn't you also let your mind wander into sexual territory as well?

Many people I speak with feel there must be something wrong or missing if they fantasize during sex about something sexual that 1) they have done before, 2) they haven't done before, or 3) that involves someone other than their partner turning them on. No, it just means you have a memory of what works for you and there are ways to incorporate your preferences into your current relationship.

You should worry about such fantasies if they become the only condition that enables you to be intimate and sexually turned on. You should also be concerned if your fantasy could harm someone. If this is the case, then I suggest you consult a therapist to deal with the issue. In general, men often fantasize about two things: 1) having amazing prowess and 2) doing something to drive a woman out of her mind with pleasure. Women are more likely to fantasize about three things: 1) being seduced, 2) exercising the power of her sexuality, and 3) being so desirable that a man can't resist her. For more ideas on how to initiate a fantasy with your lover, check out the Fantasy section.

328. What Is the Difference between a Fantasy and a Fetish?

A fantasy is the illusion or daydream one has about a specific experience. A fetish is an object that is required for the person to get sexually turned on; that object replaces another human being as the object of affection. For example, a man having a business lunch may get totally turned on by a woman in a short skirt and four-inch heels walking by, and fantasize about "doing her" over the hood of his waiting Mercedes while the valet watches. Whereas a fetishist, whose object of affection is a woman's shoe, would see the same woman walk by, but be turned on by the shoes themselves. If the woman were naked and shoeless on a bed in front of him, he wouldn't even blink, never mind become aroused. But if he were alone in a room with one or both of the woman's shoes, then he would probably be very excited. Other common objects that inspire fetishes include leather, latex, rubber, and feet. Fetishes in and of themselves are not bad, rather if people overindulge in one form of sexual stimulation, it can get in the way of having a healthy, connected sexual relationship with another person. It's a matter of keeping perspective. If you wish to spend your life making love to a shoe, go ahead. But don't expect the woman wearing the shoe to be pleased.

329. How Can I Introduce Fantasies into My Relationship?

First, do some personal inventory work on the feelings, reactions, and sensations that you want to experience. To further create your custom-made fantasies, be specific about the feeling you want to evoke. Do you want to dominate him? Do you want her to "instruct" you? For example, a woman fantasizes about receiving great oral sex from her man. She can have this played out by being the naughty school girl who is taught a "lesson" about her body by her teacher, generally referred to as a submission fantasy. A man might imagine himself as a store window model for how to play an encounter out (exhibitionism). Or you might fantasize about having group sex and becoming part of a sex-club daisy chain.

Once you know what kind of experience you want to have, then just about any idea can be adjusted to fit your needs:

1. Being dominated/submissive—master/slave (many Halloween costumes have opened doors on this particular fantasy), school teacher/ student, judge/prisoner (perhaps the bad boy prisoner has to satisfy the domineering judge).

2. Being watched or watching—voyeurism/exhibitionism.

3. Being seduced or romanced.

4. Being so sexually hot he or she can't stay away from you.

5. Group sex, multiple partners.

And whatever your personal choice may be, the real heat of role-play/ fantasies are the emotional feelings you want to evoke. And you need not dress up, although that often enhances the mood. Should explicit language be your choice, any scenario can lend itself to its use.

Once you have an idea of what gets you aroused and what scenario might elicit that arousal, then let your partner know there is something you'd love to try with him or her. To heighten the idea, you may consider starting this conversation in the morning or when you are not in the bedroom, to give both of your imaginations more time to build up anticipation. Also, name your source, as that is likely going to be your partner's first question, "What brought this up?" Tell your lover the steamy scene in a film, such as the scene with Diane Lane and Olivier Martinez in *Unfaithful*. Or tell him or her something the two of you have done before and then add the new idea in. For instance, "The last time you washed my hair, I wanted you to . . ." You can find ideas in many places—check out some of the suggestions for erotic books and movies, which are great sources for fantasy.

330. How Can I Be Sure I Taste Okay for Oral Sex? I'm Afraid for My Boyfriend to Go Down on Me Because I Think My Scent Will Turn Him Off. What Should I Do?

Good health, cleanliness, and good grooming are the number-one ways to ensure that you will taste okay. And before you assume you don't taste or smell okay, why don't you ask your partner what he thinks? If you are too nervous to ask him, then try doing a personal taste test to see how *you* actually taste. All you need to do is insert your fingers vaginally and taste the secretions. Generally, most women tend to have a naturally slightly lemony taste. If you notice a fishy smell, then you may have bacterial vaginosis; if you notice a thick, white discharge, then you may have a yeast infection. Either of these two situations can lead some women to smell a bit strong. FYI: women will often develop a yeast infection after undergoing antibiotic treatment for a situation unrelated to anything sexual. If you suspect you may have an infection, then I suggest you get checked by a trained professional; if you self-diagnose and then use an over-the-counter medication, you often prolong the problem because of an incorrect self-diagnosis. Another thing to keep in mind: a woman's scent changes throughout her cycle in reaction to vitamins, medications, or the food she eats.

331. I Worry That My Semen Tastes Too Strong. How Can I Be Sure?

Men can do the same taste test after they have masturbated—although his taste test is best done outside the shower with a hand catch instead of using a sock or towel. To adjust taste, there are two components: your natural chemistry in combination with your diet and fluid intake. Women have said men who often drink coffee or beer tend to taste more bitter; men who eat more protein tend to be "gummier" and vegetarians tend to taste "lighter." Both sexes can tell from genital secretions if their partner has been smoking. Women can tell if a man has been doing cocaine and drinking by the taste of his ejaculate. Some women and men swear by the following to "lighten" their taste: pineapple juice, fruits such as melons, kiwi, and celery. Avoid cruciferous vegetables such as cauliflower or broccoli, and for many asparagus is a major no-no. Also, if one of you is having some highly seasoned or spicy food, the other must have some as well; to quote a Hungarian woman "Your chemistries must blend."

332. My Partner Has Trouble Remaining Erect While He Is Pleasuring Me. What Can I Do?

There isn't a lot you can do until it is your turn to concentrate on him. If while concentrating on you he loses some of the rigidity of his erection, that is to be expected and your partner is very normal in this regard. Erections during lovemaking are a bit like the phases of the moon: they wax and wane, cycling between semi-erect and fully erect depending on the type of stimulation and direct attention. Let us not be held hostage by the perception that a man has to remain ramrod stiff continuously during a lovemaking session. If he is pleasuring you orally, chances are he is lying on the bed and compressing his erection and not getting any physical stimulation at the same time; both of these events would contribute to losing some volume of his erection. As soon as your attention is turned back to him and you are stimulating him directly by whatever method you choose, he will return to being fully erect.

333. How Can I Get My Wife to Go Down on Me More Often?

I am going to answer this question assuming she already enjoys giving you oral sex occasionally. For the ladies in the audience, I will tell you what men have often shared with me, "There is no such thing as too much oral sex." But I do want to clarify that men see oral sex as *part* of the lovemaking event, not its whole. What he so likes about oral sex is the heat, moisture, and softness of your mouth around his penis. "It feels so amazing." And for the gentlemen in the audience, women would "go down on you" more regularly if they knew fellatio was an interlude in sex rather than the main event. The reason women are hesitant to engage in this activity is the assumption that it will be the main event, resulting in sore jaws, sore mouth, and/or gagging. It also means that once you orgasm, you won't be having intercourse. If you know she worries about you ejaculating in her mouth, let her know with a signal when you are about to come, so she can prepare you and herself for completion. It should always be up to her whether she spits, swallows, or pulls away.

334. How Can I Achieve a G Spot Orgasm?

As Dr. Beverly Whipple (the scientist who named the G spot in recognition of Dr. Ernst Grafenberg) told me, women can find and stimulate their G spots by locating the dime-size area felt through the vaginal wall. The G spot is governed by the pelvic/hypogastric nerve system and feels different from the sensations created by the pudendal nerve system that enervates the clitoral area; also, because it is felt through the vaginal wall, it requires firmer stimulation for arousal.

The best way to achieve a G spot orgasm is after you have been highly aroused; for some women this means once they have already orgasmed. That way you will already be sexually stimulated and the tissue area of the G spot will be engorged (swollen) with blood and more easily felt. You may be able to feel the area more easily with rear-entry, doggie-style penetration, as that has the head of the man's glans stroke firmly over the already engorged G spot area, or if you are lying on top of him. If you are using fingers or a toy, the most important thing is to maintain firm-variable pressure, and use your finger in a come-here motion on the designated area. The stimulated area will have a different texture than the surrounding tissue, often more ridgy. It will range in size from a dime to a quarter. At first it may feel like you need to uri-nate, which makes sense as the area lies along the urethra. As with all sexual and physiological experiences, it often takes a number of at-tempts to narrow down whether or not something works for you. Also, know that for some women this is an off-the-charts move; for others, you might as well put them in a cold shower—it does nothing.

335. I'd Really Like to Have Anal Sex More Often. How Can I Convince My Girlfriend/Boyfriend to Do It? Also, Why Are People So Interested in Anal Sex?

First, you should know there are four possible combinations for anal sex: women and men who have been asked to receive anal penetration from their partners and women and men who have been asked to per-form anal penetration on their partners. Just in case you're thinking that there is no way a straight man is into this, I can assure you that there are many totally straight men who are interested in exploring anal play—otherwise we would have no explanation for the growing popu-larity and demand for the *Bend Over Boyfriend* I and II video tapes.

If she is interested, it's often an easier subject for a woman to broach. However, there are some men who feel that either wanting to give or receive anal sex means they have homosexual "tendencies." Let me be clear on this point: A curiosity about or an enjoyment of giving or receiving anal sex will not make anyone homosexual—male or fe-male. Nor does an interest in anal sex mean you are a latent anything—that's rubbish. Any man who is homosexual or bisexual usually knows this about his sexuality long before the topic of anal play comes up. And finally, the idea that anal play has any connection to homosexual-ity is proven clearly false by the mere fact that many women love to be anally penetrated by their men.

For those who have never explored this erotic area, a common question is, "Why?" The simple answer is that the anal area is highly sensitive. Additionally: 1) this area has a high concentration of nerves;

2) the lips on our mouths are one end of the GI tract (gastro-intestinal) and the anus is at the other end. Since we know how sensitive our lips are to sensory stimulation, we can make the deduction that the anal region is equally as sensitive; 3) During preorgasmic contractions as well as during orgasmic contractions themselves, the anal sphincters rhythmically contract. When there is something (inserted) that provides resistance, such as a penis, anal toy, or harnessed dildo, the recipient experiences an increase in sensation.

People become curious about anal sex for a couple of different reasons: 1) they see it depicted in adult films and they find it interesting and/or 2) they know their partner enjoys anal penetration. As a regular practice in heterosexual relationship, anal sex is more common outside of the U.S.

For those of you interested in either giving or receiving anal penetrative sex, you do need to know that there are two sphincters in the anus—one under voluntary control, which you can relax yourself, and one under involuntary control, which requires a form of dilation—either via a finger or a toy. So it's best to manually relax the anus before any penetration; a good rule of thumb I've been told is to use one finger for one minute and two fingers for two minutes to get the one sphincter to relax enough to have penetration and for intercourse to feel enjoyable. As a top OB-GYN has suggested, you will need to use generous amounts of water-based lubricant given the delicate tissue of this area and the fact that it is not self-lubricating.

336. If She/He Wants to Use Toys, What Does That Mean?

It means she/he has discovered new things to incorporate and make your sex life more fun. It does not mean you are not enough or enjoyable or that you no longer turn your lover on. To the contrary, a lover's desire to play with sexual toys means that he or she has a higher than normal comfort factor with you and wants to take your sex life to a different level of exploration.

337. What Is the Normal Amount of Sex per Week? My Husband Wants It at Least Once a Day and I'm Too Tired.

This is a question that only the two people in the couple can answer; there isn't a standard answer. For some couples, four times a week is just right and for others four times a month works. What I will say is that for the majority of men, when they are having sex on a regular basis, their world works better. More than one man has said regular sex with his spouse grounds him. For the majority of women who are mothers, sex will often take a backseat in priorities because they are so busy and exhausted. Sex can start to feel like just another chore to perform. This is a question that will always lead to countless magazine articles and studies, yet the truly hard facts are what works for you and your partner.

338. At What Age Do I Speak to My Children about Sex?

Sooner than you think. And rather than thinking I'll wait until age _____, don't wait. Otherwise, your children will be educated by their equally ill-informed peers and the media. There is one main thing parents want to do well—parent. There is one thing that preteens and adolescents want to do—grow up. And what is one of the biggest bastions of being an "adult"? Being sexual. The attitude of adolescents trying all that is ahead of them is as predictable as the seasons. In the face of such a fact of life is one of the more delicate formative discussions parents can have with their children, so please, oh please do not merely say, "Don't . . ." We all know how effective that was for us. Rather than say "Don't do it!", try to relate an experience with, "I wish someone had told me this was how I'd feel" or "I wish someone had warned my friend about such and such." If you have given them a responsible value system, your children will rely on those values throughout their lives and that includes the minefield known as adolescence.

339. What Is Female Ejaculation?

Before I describe the physiological sexual response called "female ejaculation," I would be remiss if I did not set one part of this straight from the get-go. It is not a true ejaculation, for it is not a muscular contraction resulting in an expulsion of a fluid. The fluid from the paraurethral (on the side of the urethra) glands is ejected in a flow, squirt, or gush of fluid typically just before orgasm. The paraurethral glands and Bartholin glands act more like a salivary gland at the moment of expulsion. People who have tasted female ejaculate say that is has a taste unto to itself; some women taste sweet, others buttery. Women who have experienced this have said there is an all-over bearing-down feeling and a sensation like a need to urinate. It can be initiated by kissing, oral sex, G spot stimulation, or intercourse.

340. Do All Women Ejaculate?

Spaniard Francisco Santa Maria Cabello, one of the foremost researchers on female ejaculation, estimates from his studies that 70 percent of all women ejaculate a fluid from the urethra that is chemically different from urine. Now, that could mean occasionally, all the time, or only once. Of those women who do so, many regularly and proactively position a towel under their hips during sex. He also states that the reason most women are not aware of the fluid is that the amount is so small it is assumed to be part of the normally heightened vaginal secretions that accompany sexual excitation. The increased exposure of this totally normal physical response of some women has resulted in the porn industry developing another "new" market niche to exploit—hence the line of videos showcasing "squirters." On the plus side, this emerging market has resulted in a general response of "Oh, thank God I'm not the only one." Some women feel more validated. On the downside, the idea that some women are "squirters" has resulted in couples feeling pressure to achieve yet another sexual goal.

341. How Do I Suggest a New Position?

First, *do not* say you did it with someone else. If it is a variation on a theme of something you already do, consider assuming the "position" and then ask to have it repeated. Successful suggestions for new-idea sources are: illustrated books, videos, scenes from films, something a friend said he or she had tried and which sounded so good that you wanted to try it. Note: None of the aforementioned sources is about a personal experience.

342. Why Does My Girlfriend Use a Vibrator?

Because it is fast and quick—after all, no man is capable of creating 50,000 oscillations per minute. Now, having said that, rest assured, gentlemen, that for most women nothing will ever replace the feel of a man's body. In much the same way, your hand may feel great, but is no comparison to a woman's body. And should you be concerned about feeling left out while she does herself with a vibrator or other toy, do what most men do with electronic equipment and ask to take over the controls.

343. Will Using a Vibrator Desensitize Her to My Touch?

If she is able to climax from other stimulation, then she has already laid down a nerve response pathway. If she uses a vibrator exclusively, it may require her weaning herself off of its intensity.

344. Where Do I Find Sex Toys?

Just about anywhere, but feel free to consult the Resource List at the back of this book. However, let me give a few pearls of wisdom. Do not order from work; using a work computer for matters of a personal nature has been grounds for dismissal. When you order from any site/ store or catalogue, ask if they sell their database. If they do, think twice about placing your order. You will end up getting a steady stream of solicitations you may very well not want your entire household to see. Also, those stores and Web sites included in the source pages have been checked out by Lou Paget's group, and if they represented that they do sell their database/mailing list, you are notified in our listings.

345. Will Toys Ever Interfere with Our Sex Life?

Only if you make the use of them the focus, not an addition, to your sexual pleasure. If toys become about performance rather than a means of exploration for your enjoyment, they can begin to interfere with your intimacy, and only the two of you know what your boundaries are. One thirty-something mother in Beverly Hills said, "It makes me crazy when my husband brings home a new toy every time he travels, which is often. I got to the point that I felt I was a lab rat being put into a testing room. When I finally told him I just wanted him, he told me his fear was I would leave if he didn't make our sex life amazing, new, and woo-woo. I almost died when he revealed this, but given our twenty-five year age difference—he's older—it made sense. But I could honestly tell him that I want only him, love handles and all. We still have an incredible collection of goodies, but now we focus on us, not on what's new."

346. I Would Really Love to Have My Wife Swallow When She Gives Me Oral Sex; How Should I Broach the Subject?

Is this a fantasy or has she done it before? If it is a fantasy, don't tell her "'cause it's so hot, baby." That will inform her that it's about someone else or you watching adult material. A better approach in this case is to tell her how it makes you feel accepted by her as a man. In both scenarios, a more moving comment to a woman is an honest statement of the impact on you as a man about how powerful it is to feel she is accepting one of the most masculine parts of you in her mouth. Corny, perhaps, but likely an easier sell than "I love seeing my seed in your mouth." And my final point: It is her mouth and only she knows if and when she is comfortable to swallow.

347. My Husband Wants to Watch Erotic Movies Together; Does That Mean There Is Something Wrong with Our Sex Life?

No. It could mean a number of things, and cheers to him for saying he wants to watch them with you. This is likely his way of opening up the conversation about what he'd like to try, however clumsily that conversation overture may have been handled. Assuming you are there with him as an audience of two, you can obviously make your choices as well.

348. Is It Normal for Him to Masturbate?

As long as his masturbating is an adjunct to your sex life and not his sole outlet to exclusion of you. I would hazard a guess that since he tells you about his masturbation and does not try to hide it, he is comfortable with this as a natural part of his sexual life. Most men, including those who are married, happy, and sexually active with their wives, masturbate regularly—some rarely, some often. Many men say that masturbation is less a sexual act and more a physical release. Some women ask if it is different if their man masturbates in the shower versus in front of a porn film. My response is no, not necessarily. The important point to remember is whether or not the masturbation is done to your exclusion or to avoid having sex with you.

349. We Used to Have a Great Sex Life, How Do We Get the Spark Back?

Do you want it back? If so, do not expect anyone other than you to deliver it. If the spark was there before, it is still there, perhaps turned down, but still there nonetheless. In the beginning, when you were planning to be together, you made being together a priority and planned for it. How do you spell "date night" in America? I feel a bit like a broken record in this regard, but there are two main reasons for the lack of spark/intimacy for couples: 1) no time and 2) being tired. This sad state of affairs is especially true for parents. Couples whom I have seen work at keeping their sexual connection going do so with intention and planning. They do not take for granted that sex is going to happen out of thin air; they still plan for it—twenty years after their vows. They may be more accessible physically to each other, but that does not mean they take a great sex life for granted. For the parents: one must be very organized and a better planner. Check out Tips 147, 159, and 175 for ideas on how to plan for sex when you're parents.

350. Viagra Is Not for Everyone.

Although many men have experienced and reported positive results with the use of Viagra, enabling them to attain erections and last longer,

Viagra is not for every man. The product Web site provides these cautions: "For patients with preexisting cardiovascular disease, sexual activity may present a cardiac risk. VIAGRA has mild and transient vasodilatory effects. Physicians should consider the impact of resuming sexual activity and the vasodilatory effects of VIAGRA on patients before initiating treatment. Patients with . . . recent serious cardiovascular events, hypotension or uncontrolled hypertension, or retinitis pigmentosa did not participate in preapproval clinical trials. In these patients, physicians should prescribe VIAGRA with caution."

Further, the Web site stated that "the most common side effects of VIAGRA were headache (16 percent), flushing (10 percent), and dyspepsia (7 percent). Adverse events, including visual effects (3 percent), were generally transient and mild to moderate."

351. Great Lover Moment: Don't Listen to Certain Stats.

A woman who recently attended one of my seminars voiced a common anxiety I hear from women: "Am I sexually dysfunctional if I don't orgasm all the time?" I think her concern is directly related to the much-publicized statistic that came out a couple of years ago that 43 percent of women are sexually dysfunctional. This statistic is completely misleading, as Dr. Leonore Tiefer pointed out in a 1999 study. The 43 percent stat was based on an incomplete and cursory poll done in 1994, and yet the number was widely bandied about by the media, making women across the country question their sexual functioning. In her book with Ellyn Kaschak, Ph.D., *A New View of Women's Sexual Problems*, Dr. Tiefer says that the medical establishment does not begin to represent women's sexuality, the problems they are experiencing, or their causes. In the wake of this "new myth," Dr. Tiefer has spearheaded a new organization called FSD-Alert.org (FSD is female sexual dysfunction), to look at how women's sexuality should be studied and understood.

352. The Skinny on Pheromones.

We've all heard talk about the power of pheromones, chemicals released by the brain and body, to communicate sexual attraction or interest between males and females. And while most of these studies are based on animals and insects, recent technology has been able to measure the effect of pheromones between humans. However, within the scientific community, questions remain as to whether or not we actually communicate with one another at this level. Studies in the 1980s by Martha McClintock, a professor of psychology at the University of Chicago, showed how pheromones helped to synchronize ovulation and menstruation of women who live together. Now new research indicates that men exposed to the chemicals a woman secretes when she is ovulating observe a spike in testosterone levels. The researcher, Astrid Juette, a psychologist at the University of Vienna in Austria, said her work was the "first time that someone has shown that men differentiate between women at different stages of their menstrual cycles." However, some scientists still question whether we really do respond to the pheromones of others. "Human vomeronasal organs (VNO) channel these odors from the nasal passages to the limbic system, but how, they argue, are these odors received and to what end?" From *Contemporary Sexuality*, Vol. 36, No. 12, Dec 2002.

353. Alabama and Sex Toys.

An Alabama law criminalizing the sale of sex toys was deemed unconstitutional in October 2002. In a district court ruling, the 1998 Anti-Obscenity Enforcement Act was tossed out for being "unnecessarily intrusive," as reported by *Contemporary Sexuality* (Vol. 36, No. 11, Nov 2002). Why would they need to ban sex toys? Too many people having too much fun?

354. Infants Like Leather?

New research indicates that "leather clothing as an accessory to sexual activity may have its roots in skin eroticism." Skin eroticism begins in infancy, with the mother's caressing touch of an infant, helping the baby become sensitive to the sensual world within and without. Further "clinical evidence suggests that such pleasurable physical interactions [with the mother] help to immunize the child against the future development of body and gender dissatisfaction and are also crucial to the development of a coherent, integrated body image" (Provence & Lipton, 1962). *Contemporary Sexuality*, Vol. 36, No. 11, Nov 2002.

355. The Truth about Circumcision.

In this country, circumcision is largely performed in hospitals, by medical personnel, but its origins are decidedly religious and cultural. Extending before Jesus' apparent circumcision (Luke 2:21) and referred to directly in the Old Testament, "Every male shall be circumcised. You shall be circumcised in the flesh of your foreskin, and it shall be a sign of the covenant between me and you" (Genesis 17:10–11). But the roots of this increasingly contentious procedure reach far deeper into the past than just two millennia. Depicted in ancient Egyptian bas reliefs, circumcision has been called by some a form of social control or a mark of cultural identity like a tattoo or body piercing. But the surgery didn't become routine among American medical practitioners until the late nineteenth century. Today, it's the sensation of pain at the time of male circumcision—and a perceived loss of sexual pleasure in the decades after the surgery—that has given rise to an anticircumcision movement in the U.S. Organized efforts to change attitudes and policy toward the surgery began soon after the American Academy of Pediatrics (AAP) Committee on the Fetus and Newborn declared in 1971 that "there was no valid medical indication for circumcision in the neonatal period." In the mid-1970s, four out of every five males in the U.S. had been circumcised. Today, the rate has fallen to 61 percent. *Contemporary Sexuality*, Vol. 36, No. 10, Oct 2002.

356. Smoking and Teenage Sex.

Of all risky behavior, parental smoking is most closely associated with teenage sexual activity according to a study published in *The Milbank Quarterly*, a health-care policy journal. The survey of 19,000 youths in grades seven through twelve found that adolescents whose parents smoked were 50 percent more likely than children of nonsmokers to report having had sex, and more of them report having had sex before age fifteen. "I think that parents who smoke provide a model of unsafe behavior and create an atmosphere where it's okay to live on the edge," said Dr. Esther Wilder, as assistant professor of sociology at Lehmann College and author of the study. (*The New York Times*, 9/3/02.)

357. Seniors and Sex.

Recent research on the sex life of seniors has illuminated what was once rarely thought of, much less asked about. AARP/*Modern Maturity* Sexuality Study, conducted in 1999, found that 44 percent of women and half of men seventy-five years and older believe that "a satisfying sexual relationship" is important to their quality of life. That said, half or less of all those 75 years old or older were "very" or "somewhat" satisfied with their sex lives, indicating that a lot of them are less satisfied. But one caveat was posed by sexual educator Peggy Brick, "one of my concerns is there seems to be a push in the sexology community that older people are very sexual. It's very genitally focused. Some may not be, in terms of having intercourse." It may simply mean touching or cuddling. *Contemporary Sexuality*, Vol. 36, No. 9, Sept 2002.

358. HPV Less in Circumcised Men.

A study published in *The New England Journal of Medicine* suggests that circumcised men are less likely to infect their female partners with the human papilloma virus (HPV) than uncircumcised men with poor hygiene in instances in which the men have had six or more partners. Further, certain strains of HPV (numbers 16 and 18) are associated with cervical cancer in women. *Contemporary Sexuality*, Vol. 36, No. 5, May 2002.

359. Virtual Reality Sex.

An Australian inventor has a new way for long-distance lovers to engage in sex: virtual reality sex. Dominic Choy of New South Wales is attempting to patent his online computer technology, reports *New Scientist* magazine. The two lovers don virtual reality visors from wherever they are and use touch and sound sensors to issue signals to their partners across the globe. The technology also allows participants to alter the appearance of their virtual partners, transforming their images, for instance, into that of their favorite celebrity. This added feature may interfere, so watch those celebrity fantasies. Reuters, January 17, as quoted in *Contemporary Sexuality*, Vol. 35, No. 2, Feb 2001.

360. Fantasies Worldwide.

Erotic fantasies fill the minds of three-quarters of people on the globe, but less than half ever act them out according to a poll released by Harlequin Enterprises, a publisher of romantic books. South America led in fantasy thinking with 95 percent of Argentinians and Chileans admitting to an active fantasy life. Japan came in last, with only one out of two people acknowledging their wandering minds. Reuters, January 16—polled 5,000 men and women.

361. Chastity Belts Are Back, Sort Of.

Several companies are selling modern versions of the medieval device on the Internet. In both the Middle Ages and the twenty-first century, the purpose of the chastity belt is to prevent the wearer from having sex with anyone else—regardless of whether the belt is used seriously or not. Made of plastic, so it doesn't set off metal detectors, the new chastity belt costs $159.95 and weighs five ounces and comes in hot pink. Oh, and one more thing, these are made for men! *Contemporary Sexuality,* Vol. 35, No. 6, June 2001.

362. Intersex: More Common Than Cystic Fibrosis.

"ISNA (Intersex Society of North America) estimates that about 1 in every 2,000 babies is born with an intersex condition, based on the number of newborns referred to 'gender identity teams' in major hospitals. At this frequency, intersex (formerly referred to as hermaphroditism, a term ISNA wants to ban) is more common than cystic fibrosis, whose incidence is about 1 in 2,300 live births. Intersex people are born with 'ambiguous, outsized or tiny genitalia' making their gender indetermined—most boys with 'tiny' penises were made into girls by cutting off the penis, and most girls with 'outsized' genitalia were cut because the clitoris was seen as 'too big.'" Intersex means that "'a person with an intersex condition has some parts usually associated with males and some parts usually associated with females, or that she or he has some parts that appear ambiguous (like a phallus that looks somewhere between a penis and a clitoris, or a divided scrotum that looks more like a labia).'" From *Fathering Magazine*, November 20, 2002 as reprinted in *Contemporary Psychology,* December 2002.

363. Sex As Prevention.

Sex twice a week may prevent the common cold, say researchers at Wilkes University, Pennsylvania. After studying the sex habits of undergraduate students, researchers concluded that students who had sex once or twice a week had one third more immunoglobulin A (IgA) in their saliva. Elevated levels of IgA protect us from colds, flu, and other infections. Surprisingly, more sex is not better. Researchers found that those students who had sex more than three times per week had lower IgA levels than those who rarely had sex or had no sex at all. Moderation seems to be the key. *Healthy Immunity*, newsletter.

364. Birth Control Pills and Vitamin Depletion.

Birth control pills have been seen to deplete a woman's body of vitamin C, B12, B2, folic acid and magnesium. If you're on the pill, make sure that you take a vitamin supplement. *Drug Induced Nutrient Depletion Handbook*, Morton Publishing Co.

365. Birth Control: The Choices Expand.

Sterilization, birth control pills, and the male condom are the most widely used forms of birth control in the U.S. But researchers are promising "a new era in birth control" options, with many new forms being introduced in upcoming months. According to a recent WNBC. com gathering of information, here is a listing of those currently available:

- **Reality female condom**—sold without a prescription, it is a lubricated polyurethane sheath that is slipped, closed-end first, into the vagina. The open end remains outside, partially covering the labia. The Reality is held in place internally by an adjustable, small diaphragm-like ring at the end. A favorite for couples who want anal protection because of the size and strength of the polyurethane. For anal use, one merely slips out the position ring.

- **Diaphragms**—available by prescription and sized by a health professional for proper fit. Women apply a spermicide before inserting it until the dome-shaped disk covers the cervix.

- **Cervical cap**—available by prescription and sized and used similarly to a diaphragm.

- **Depo-Provera**—a contraceptive hormone injection given by a health professional every three months.

- **IUDs**—T-shaped devices inserted into the uterus by a health professional that work for up to one year, five years, or ten years, depending on the type.

- **Vaginal spermicides**—available without prescription in foam, cream, jelly, film, suppository, or tablet forms. The active ingredient in spermicides, nonoxynol-9, has been shown to be very irritating to some women and men.

- **Preven kits**—a collection of morning-after pills and a pregnancy test. This emergency contraception may prevent pregnancy up to three days after unprotected sex.

- **Lunelle**—a contraceptive hormone injection given by a health professional every month.

- **Nuvaring**—a flexible, polymer, vaginal ring that a woman wears three weeks a month to prevent pregnancy. It releases a continuous, low dose of a combination of estrogen and progestin hormones.

- **Ortho Evra**—the first birth control patch, worn three weeks of the month. The weekly application of the thin 1¾" square delivers a consistent transdermal dosage of estrogen and progestin.

- **Essure**—a tiny, springlike device that is inserted into a woman's fallopian tubes, where it causes scar tissue to grow and permanently plug the tubes.

Whatever your choice of birth control, make that choice in an informed manner and in a way that fits your lifestyle. The Today Sponge is also coming back into production in Canada in April 2003.

Resources

Where You Can Get the Toys

In collecting the best sources for toy products, I asked store owners several questions in order to verify their commitment to quality and an open, encouraging attitude: Did they have a positive sex attitude? Would a woman be comfortable going into the store by herself or ordering over the phone? How big was the store's selection? Did they sell their mailing list? Was their Web site secure?

Catalogs are a great, safe way to introduce tools into the relationship. The very act of choosing a toy can be a bonding, intimate experience. It's a gentle way of suggesting to your partner what you'd like to try sexually. By looking at the pictures together, you and your partner can feel each other out about what may seem like fun, what may seem too risky, and so on. Initially, making suggestions can make you feel vulnerable. Women, especially, fear being rejected. Remember, gentlemen, they don't want to risk being perceived as "loose," if they suggest using a sex toy.

Essentially, the catalogs I am recommending are tasteful. A couple of these outfits are more oriented toward women, all provide wonderful support staff to answer questions via an 800 number, and all have careful explanations in the catalogs themselves. Other catalogs are a bit more edgy and less pristine. (And be aware: Adam & Eve sells its mailing list.)

Condomania
www.condomania.com
Order line: 800-9CONDOMS (926-6367)

This Web site and phone/mail order service is one of the best nonretail sources for condoms. The Web site uses SSL encryption for placing orders.

The West

SEATTLE

Toys in Babeland
707 East Pike St., Seattle WA 98122
206-328-2914 / Catalog: 800-658-9119
E-mail: *biglove@babeland.com* / Web site: *www.babeland.com*

This is a female-run store, originally created as a place for women and their comfort. It now carries some male-oriented products. Workshops and seminars are also offered.

RENO

Romantic Sensations
1055 S Virginia Street, Reno NV 89502
775-322-1884

Ten thousand square feet of just about every product imaginable. Experienced sales staff.

San Francisco

Good Vibrations

Retail stores:
1210 Valencia St., San Francisco CA 94110
2502 San Pablo Ave., Berkeley CA 94702

Mail order:
938 Howard St., Suite 101, San Francisco CA 94103
415-974-8990
Fax: 415-974-8989 / E-mail: *goodvibe@well.com*
Web site: *www.goodvibes.com*

Good Vibrations is one of the best all-around store/catalog combinations. All their products have passed customer satisfaction tests. The staff is known for its courteous, nonjudgmental, sex-positive attitude, and knowledgable service.

Sacramento

Mystique Boutique
328 D Street, Marysville CA 95901 (40 miles north of Sacramento)
530-743-6449

Carries a wide range of toys as well as lubricants. Very friendly staff.

Santa Cruz

Hot Stuff
56 N Saratoga Ave., Santa Clara CA 95051
408-241-9971

Two separate stores, one offering toys and novelties, the other offering a wide range of videos and DVDs for every taste. Something for everyone!

LOS ANGELES

The Pleasure Chest
7733 Santa Monica Blvd., Los Angeles CA 90046
323-650-1022 / Order line: 800-753-4536
Fax: 323-650-1176 / Web site: *www.thepleasurechest.com*

This Pleasure Chest targets a primarily gay male clientele, with a strong leather focus, though straight men and women will find many products for them, including videos and apparel.

The Love Boutique
18637 Ventura Blvd., Tarzana CA 91356
818-342-2400
2924 Wilshire Blvd., Santa Monica CA 90403
310-453-3459 / Toll-free ordering: 888-568-4663

The two stores are female-owned and operated and are open seven days a week. The staff seems uniquely focused on making women feel more at ease and comfortable with their sexuality.

REDWOOD CITY

Ultimate Elegance
733 El Camino Real, Redwood City CA 94063
650-369-6913 / Website: *www.ultimatelegance.com*

They test the products themselves, and won't carry items that don't work.

San Diego

F Street Stores (five stores in the San Diego area)

751 Fourth Ave., San Diego CA 92101 / 619-236-0841
2004 University Ave, San Diego CA 92104 / 619-298-2644
7998 Miramar Rd., San Diego CA 92126 / 619-549-8014
1141 Third Ave., Chula Vista CA 92011 / 619-585-3314
237 East Grand, Escondido CA 92023 / 619-480-6031

The stores in this chain offer a wide range of male- and female-oriented products; it was also one of the first to create a women's novelty section.

Condoms Plus
1220 University Ave., San Diego CA 92103
619-291-7400

This is a store "with a woman in mind." It is a general license store for all sorts of gifts, as well as condoms. In other words, you can buy a stuffed animal for your child as well as an adult novelty item for your husband. The novelties, however, are in their own section of the store.

Utah

Jack n' Jills
4421 Harrison Depot, Ogden UT 84403
801-476-1680

Clean, friendly store with helpful staff.

The Midwest

CHICAGO

The Pleasure Chest (affiliated with the store in New York)
3155 North Broadway, Chicago IL 60657
773-525-7152 / Catalog sales: 800-316-9222
www.pleasurechesttoys.com

The majority of customers are women and couples. This is the store that defined what an adult store should be like: clean, bright, tastefully presented, with nonjudgmental salespeople who are like you and me. This and the New York store show the impact of being run and operated by the owner, who focuses on taking good care of the customer.

Frenchy's
872 North State St., Chicago IL 60610
312-337-9190

This store has undergone a major renovation in appearance and size. It is now three times larger and offers a range of products for men and women.

MINNEAPOLIS/ST. PAUL

Fantasy House Gifts
769 West Lake St., Minneapolis MN 55408
612-824-2459 / Web site: *www.fantasygifts.com*

There are eight Fantasy House stores in the area, including Bloomington, Bernsville, St. Louis Park, Crystal, Fridley, Coon Rapids, and St. Paul— and two stores in New Jersey: in Marlton and Turnersville. Adult material and novelties presented with a comfortable Midwestern environment and attitude.

OKLAHOMA

Christies Toy Box
1184 North MacArthur Blvd., Oklahoma City OK 73127
405-942-4622

Christies is part of a chain of adult stores, ranked number one in the state of Oklahoma; stores also exist in Texas.

WISCONSIN

A Woman's Touch
600 Williamson St., Madison WI 53703
888-621-8880 or 608-250-1928 / Web site:
www.touchofawoman.com

Newsletter posted on site with seminars and workshops. Books and videos prescreened to be sure they are female friendly. Site encrypted. Run by an M.D. and M.S.W. (social worker) and featuring very current information updates.

The East

CONNECTICUT

Naughty Nancy's
60 Connecticut Ave., Norwalk CT 06850
203-866-7175 / 888-44-NANCY (888-446-2629)
Web site: *www.naughtynancys.com*

Owner takes pride in having a woman-friendly store that's not sleazy. Great sense of humor and knowledgable about the products being offered.

MAINE

Midnight Boutique
571 Main Street, Lewiston ME 04240
207-753-0443

Clean, well-run store with knowledgable sales staff ready to assist you.

NEW YORK

The Pleasure Chest
156 Seventh Ave. South (between Charles and Perry),
 New York NY 10014
212-242-4185 / Catalog sales: 800-316-9222
New York store customer service: 800-643-1025
Web site: *www.pleasurechesttoys.com*

The New York store and its Chicago sister store are both popular, classy, and well-stocked, with a range of products for both men and women, straight and gay.

Eve's Garden
119 West 57th St., Suite 1201, New York NY 10019
212-757-8651 / Orders: 800-848-3837
Web site: *www.evesgarden.com*

This is a female-owned and operated store. What the Pleasure Chest did in 1972 for gay male consumers, Eve's Garden did for women in 1974. Located in the heart of midtown Manhattan, Eve's Garden is in the least likely of areas. It is known far and wide as the matriarch of feminine-focused, sex-positive merchandising.

Toys in Babeland
94 Rivington St., New York NY 10002
212-375-1701 / E-mail: *comments@babeland.com*
Web site: *www.babeland.com*

New York branch of the Seattle-based operation.

The South

FLORIDA

Giggles
4407 S Tamiami Trail, Sarasota FL 34231
941-927-7474

Just about the friendliest, most well-trained staff you'd ever want to meet.

NORTH CAROLINA

Adam & Eve
PO Box 8200, Hillsborough NC 27278
800-293-4654 / Customer Service: 919-644-8100

This is the biggest mail-order adult products company in the United States. It offers a full range of products. Sells its mailing list.

Texas

Forbidden Fruit
108 E. North Loop Blvd., Austin TX 78751
512-453-8090 / Web site: *www.forbiddenfruit.com*

Three locations in Austin. Very female-friendly atmosphere. Seminars. The site is secure.

Canada

Vancouver

Womyns' Ware Inc.
896 Commercial Drive, Vancouver BC V5L 3Y5
Order desk: 888-996-9273 / Store: 604-254-2543
Web site: *www.womynsware.com*

Love Nest
119 East 1st St., North Vancouver BC V7L 1B2
604-987-1175 / Web site: *www.lovenest.ca*

Tony and Kira, the husband-wife owner-operators, just opened their second store in Whistler, BC.

Calgary

The Love Boutique
9737 MacLeod Trail SW., Calgary AB T2J 0P6
403-252-1846

Just for Lovers
920 36th St. NE, #114, Calgary AB / 403-273-6242
4014 MacLeod Trail S., Calgary AB / 403-243-2554
4247 Bow Trail SW, Calgary AB / 403-282-7125

WINNIPEG

Discreet Boutique
317 Ellis (or 340 Donald, depending on which entrance you use),
Winnipeg Manitoba R3B 2H7
204-947-1307

HALIFAX

Venus Envy
1598 Barrington St., Halifax NS B3J 1Z6
902-422-0004 / Web site: *www.venusenvy.ca*

OTTAWA

Venus Envy
110 Parent Ave., Ottawa ON K1N 7B4
613-789-4646 / Web site: *www.venusenvy.ca*

TORONTO

Seduction
577 Yonge St., Toronto ON M4Y 1Z2
416-966-6969

Fifteen thousand square feet on three floors.

Come As You Are
701 Queen Street West, Toronto ON M6J 1E6
877-858-3160 / Web site: *www.comeasyouare.com*

"Good sex is a cooperative effort." Only cooperative-run sex store in Canada.

Any of the listed products in the book can be purchased through the Sexuality Seminars/Frankly Speaking, Inc. All transactions are confidential and we do not sell our mailing list. To purchase products, inquire about Lou Paget's seminar schedule, book a seminar, be placed on the Frankly Speaking mailing list, or to get more information, call 1-877-SexSeminars (1-877-739-7364).

Purchases can be made with Visa/MasterCard, cash, or check. Frankly Speaking Inc. shows on all bank statements and is the name under which all correspondence is sent. All products are discreetly packaged and shipped Priority Post unless otherwise requested. The Specialty Sophist-Kits gift boxes can arrive in presentation style (open) or closed—for a bigger surprise. They are delivered UPS or Federal Express and are shipped through Artful Baskets.

For more information, we can be reached at:

Frankly Speaking, Inc.
11601 Wilshire Blvd., Suite 500
Los Angeles CA 90025
310-556-3623
E-mail: *office@loupaget.com* / Web site: *www.loupaget.com*

Bibliography

Anand, Margo. *The Art of Sexual Ecstasy: The Path of Sacred Sexuality for Western Lovers.* Los Angeles: Jeremy Tarcher, 1989.

Anand, Margo. *The Art of Sexual Magic: Cultivating Sexual Energy to Transform Your Life.* New York: Tarcher/Putnam, 1995.

Anand, Margo. *Sexual Ecstasy: The Art of Orgasm, Exercises from The Art of Sexual Magic.* New York: Tarcher/Putnam, 2000.

Bakos, Susan Crain. *What Men Really Want: Straight Talk from Men About Sex.* New York: St. Martin's, 1990.

Barbach, Lonnie. *For Each Other: Sharing Sexual Intimacy.* New York: Anchor Press/Doubleday, 1982.

Bechtel, Stefan. *The Practical Encyclopedia of Sex and Health.* Emmaus, Penn.: Rodale, 1993.

Bechtel, Stefan. *Sex: A Man's Guide.* Emmaus, Penn.: Rodale, 1996.

Bell, Simon, Richard Curtis, and Helen Fielding. *Who's Had Who.* New York: Warner Books, 1990.

Birch, Robert. *Oral Caress: The Loving Guide to Exciting a Woman. A Comprehensive Illustrated Manual on the Joyful Art of Cunnilingus.* Columbus, Ohio: PEC Publications, 1996.

Bishop, Clifford. *Sex and Spirit: Ecstasy and Transcendence, Ritual and Taboo, the Undivided Self.* New York: Little, Brown and Company, 1996.

Black, Jules. *Body Talk: An A–Z Guide to Women's Health.* London: Angus & Robertson Publishers, 1988.

Block, Joel D. and Susan Crain Bakos. *Sex over 50.* Paramus, New Jersey: Reward Books, 1999.

Blue, Violet, ed. *Sweetlife: Erotic Fantasies for Couples.* San Francisco: Cleis Press, 2001.

Blue, Violet, ed. *The Ultimate Guide to Cunnilingus: How to Go Down on a Woman and Give Her Exquisite Pleasure.* San Francisco: Cleis Press, 2002.

Blue, Violet, ed. *The Ultimate Guide to Adult Videos: How to Watch Adult Videos and Make Your Sex Life Sizzle.* San Francisco: Cleis Press, 2003.

Brame, Gloria. *Come Hither: A Commonsense Guide to Kinky Sex.* New York: Fireside Books, 1999.

Bright, Susie, ed. *The Best American Erotica 2003.* New York: Touchstone, 2003.

Britten, Rhonda. *Fearless Loving: 8 Simple Truths That Will Change the Way You Date, Mate, and Relate.* New York: Dutton, 2003.

Caine, K. Winston. *The Male Body: An Owner's Manual.* Emmaus, Penn.: Rodale, 1996.

Chalker, Rebecca. *The Clitoral Truth: The Secret World at Your Fingertips.* New York: Seven Stories Press, 2000.

Chang, Dr. Stephen T. *The Tao of Sexology: The Book of Infinite Wisdom.* Reno, Nev.: Tao Publishing, 1986.

Chesser, Eustace. *Strange Loves: The Human Aspects of Sexual Deprivation.* New York: William Morrow and Company, 1971.

Chia, Mantak and Douglas Abrams. *The Multi-Orgasmic Male: How Every Man Can Experience Multiple Orgasms and Dramatically Enhance His Sexual Relationship.* San Francisco: Harper, 1997.

Chia, Mantak and Maneewan Chia. *Cultivating Female Sexual Energy: Healing Love Through the Tao.* Huntington, New York: Healing Tao Books, 1986.

·Chichester, B., ed. *Sex Secrets: Ways to Satisfy Your Partner Every Time.* Emmaus, Penn.: Rodale, 1996.

Chu, Valentin. *The Yin Yang Butterfly: Ancient Chinese Sexual Secrets for Western Lovers.* New York: Tarcher/Putnam, 1993.

Cohen, Angela and Sarah Gardner Fox. *The Wise Woman's Guide to Erotic Videos: 300 Sexy Videos for Every Woman—and her Lover.* New York: Broadway, 1997.

Comfort, Alex. *The Joy of Sex: A Gourmet Guide to Lovemaking.* New York: Fireside/Simon and Schuster, 1972.

Comfort, Alex. *The New Joy of Sex: A Gourmet Guide to Lovemaking for the Nineties.* New York: Crown Publishers, Inc.,1991.

Danielou, Alain. *The Complete Kama Sutra: The First Unabridged Modern Translation of the Classic Indian Text.* Rochester, Vermont: Park Street Press, 1994.

Deida, David. *The Way of the Superior Lover: A Spiritual Guide to the Sexual Skills.* Texas: Plexus, 1997.

Dodson, Betty. *Sex For One: The Joy of Selfloving.* New York: Crown Books, 1996.

Douglas, Nik and Penny Slinger. *Sexual Secrets: The Alchemy of Ecstasy.* 10th Anniversary Issue. Rochester, Vermont: Destiny Books, 1989.

Eichel, Edward and Philip Nobile. *The Perfect Fit: How to Achieve Mutual Fulfillment and Monogamous Passion Through the New Intercourse.* New York: Signet, 1993.

Ellison, Carol Rinkleib. *Women's Sexualities: Generations of Women Share Intimate Secrets of Sexual Self-Acceptance.* Oakland, Calif.: New Harbinger, 2000.

Fisher, Helen. *Anatomy of Love: The Natural History of Monogamy, Adultery and Divorce.* New York: W.W. Norton, 1992.

Fisher, Helen. *The First Sex: The Natural Talents of Women and How They Are Changing the World.* New York: Random House, 1999.

Ganem, Marc, M.D. *La sexualite du couple pendant la grossesse: guide pratique.* Paris: Filipacchi, 1992.

George, Stephen C. *A Lifetime of Sex: The Ultimate Manual on Sex, Women and Relationships for Every Stage of a Man's Life.* Emmaus, Penn.: Rodale, 1998.

Goldstein, Irwin and Larry Rothstein. *The Potent Male*. Regenesis Cycle Press, 1995.

Gottman, John M. *The Relationship Cure: A 5-Step Guide to Strengthening Your Marriage, Family, and Friendships*. New York: Crown Publishers, 2001.

Gottman, John M. *The Seven Principles for Making Marriage Work*. New York: Crown Publishers, 1999.

Hatcher, Robert A. *Contraceptive Technology*. 16th Ed. New York: Irvington Publishers, 1994.

Hite, Shere. *The Hite Report: A Nationwide Study on Female Sexuality*. New York: Dell, 1976.

Hite, Shere. *The Hite Report: On Male Sexuality*. New York: Ballantine, 1981.

Hopkins, Martha. *Intercourses: An Aphrodisiac Cookbook*. Memphis, Tenn.: Terrace Publishing, 1997.

Janus, Samual and Cynthia Janus. *The Janus Report on Sexual Behavior: The First Broad-Scale Scientific National Survey Since Kinsey*. New York: John Wiley & Sons, 1993.

Kahn, Sandra. *The Kahn Report on Sexual Preferences*. New York: Avon, 1981.

Kaplan, Helen Singer. *The New Sex Therapy: The Active Treatment of Sexual Disorders*. New York: Brunner/Mazel, 1974.

Kaschak, Ellyn and Leonore Tiefer, eds. *A New View of Women's Sexual Problems*. Binghamton, New York: Hayworth Press, 2001.

Keesling, Barbara. *How To Make Love All Night (and Drive a Woman Wild): Male Multiple Orgasm and Other Secrets for Prolonging Lovemaking*. New York: Harper Perennial, 1994.

Keesling, Barbara. *Sexual Pleasure: Reaching New Heights of Sexual Arousal & Intimacy*. Alameda, Calif.: Hunter House, 1993.

Klein, Marty. *Beyond Orgasm: Dare to Be Honest About the Sex You Really Want*. Berkeley, Calif.: Celestial Arts, 2002.

Kline-Graber, Georgia and Benjamin Graber. *A Guide to Sexual Satisfaction: Women's Orgasm*. New York: Popular Library, 1976.

Kronhausen, Phyllis and Eberhard. *The Complete Book of Erotic Art, Vols. 1 & 2*. New York: Bell Publishing Company, 1978.

Knutila, John. *Fit For Sex: A Man's Guide to Enhancing and Maintaining Peak Sexual Performance.* Paramus, New Jersey: Reward Books, 2000.

Ladas Kahn, Alice, Beverly Whipple, and John Perry. *The G Spot: And Other Recent Discoveries About Human Sexuality.* New York: Dell, 1982.

Lee, Victoria. *Ecstatic Lovemaking: An Intimate Guide to Soulful Sex.* Berkeley, Calif.: Conari Press, 2002.

Love, Brenda. *Encyclopedia of Unusual Sex Practices.* New York: Barricade Books, 1992.

Mann, A.T., and Jane Lyle. *Sacred Sexuality.* Shaftesbury, England: Element Books Limited, 1995.

Massey, Doreen. *Lover's Guide Encyclopedia: The Definitive Guide to Sex and You.* New York: Thunder's Mouth Press, 1996.

Masters, William, Virginia Johnson, and Robert C. Kolodny. *Heterosexuality.* New York: HarperCollins, 1994.

Masters, William and Virginia Johnson. *Human Sexual Response.* Boston: Little, Brown and Company, 1966.

McGraw, Phillip C. *Relationship Rescue: A Seven Step Strategy for Reconnecting with Your Partner.* New York: Hyperion, 2000.

McCutcheon, Marc. *The Compass in Your Nose and Other Astonishing Facts About Humans.* Los Angeles: Jeremy P. Tarcher Inc., 1989.

McCary, James Leslie. *Sexual Myths and Fallacies.* New York: Schocken, 1973.

Meletis, Chris D. *Better Sex Naturally: Herbs and Other Natural Supplements that Can Jump Start Your Sex Life.* New York: Philip Lief Group, 2000.

Milsten, Richard and Julian Slowinski. *The Sexual Male: Problems and Solutions: A Complete Medical and Psychological Guide to Lifelong Potency.* New York: W.W. Norton and Company, 1999.

Mooney, Shane. *Useless Sexual Trivia: Tastefully Prurient Facts About Everyone's Favorite Subject.* New York: Fireside, 2000.

Muir, Charles and Caroline. *Tantra: The Art of Conscious Loving.* San Francisco: Mercury House, 1989.

Neret, Gilles. *Erotica Universalis.* Cologne, Germany: Benedikt Tashcen Verlag, 1994.

Ogden, Gina. *Women Who Love Sex: An Inquiry into the Expanding Spirit of Women's Erotic Experience.* Cambridge, Mass.: Womanspirit Press, 1999.

Otto, Herbert A. *Liberated Orgasms: The Orgasmic Revolution.* Silverado, Calif.: Liberating Creations, 1999.

Panati, Charles. *Sexy Origins and Intimate Things: The Rites and Rituals of Straights, Gays, Bis, Drags, Trans, Virgins, and Others.* New York: Penguin Books, 1998.

Parsons, Alexandra. *Facts & Phalluses: A Collection of Bizarre and Intriguing Truths, Legends and Measurements.* New York: St. Martin's Press, 1998.

Pearsall, Paul, Ph.D. *Super Immunity.* New York: Fawcett, 1993.

Purvis, Kenneth. *The Male Sexual Machine: An Owner's Manual.* New York: St. Martin's Press, 1992.

Ramsdale, David and Ellen. *Sexual Energy Ecstasy: A Practical Guide to Lovemaking Secrets of the East and West.* New York: Bantam, 1993.

Rancier, Lance. *The Sex Chronicles: Strange-But-True Tales from Around the World.* Los Angeles, Calif.: General Publishing Group, 1997.

Raskin, Valerie Davis. *Great Sex for Moms: Ten Steps to Nurturing Passions While Raising Kids.* New York: Fireside, 2002.

Reinsch, Judith. *The Kinsey Institute New Report on Sex: What You Must Know to Be Sexually Literate.* New York: St. Martin's Press, 1990.

Rilly, Cheryl. *Great Moments in Sex.* New York: Three Rivers Press, 1999.

Sacks, Stephen. *The Truth About Herpes,* 4th ed. Vancouver, Canada: Gordon Soules Publishers, 1997.

Schwartz, Bob and Leah Schwartz. *The One Hour Orgasm: How to Learn the Amazing 'Venus Butterfly,'* 3rd ed. Houston, Texas: Breakthru Publishing, 1999.

Smith, David and Mike Gordon. *Strange But True Facts About Sex: The Illustrated Book of Sexual Trivia.* Minnetonka, Minn.: Meadowbrook Press, 1989.

Stoppard, Miriam. *The Magic of Sex: The Book That Really Tells Men About Women and Women About Men.* New York: Dorling Kindersley, 1991.

Stubbs, Kenneth Ray and Saulnier. *Erotic Massage: The Touch of Love.* Larkspur, Calif.: Secret Garden, 1993.

Stubbs, Kenneth. *The Essential Tantra: A Modern Guide to Sacred Sexuality.* New York: Jeremy Tarcher, 1999.

Taormino, Tristan. *The Ultimate Guide to Anal Sex for Women.* San Francisco: Cleis Press, 1998.

Tannahill, Reay. *Sex in History.* Briarcliff Manor, New York: Scarborough House, 1980.

Tannen, Deborah. *You Just Don't Understand: Women and Men in Conversation.* New York: William Morrow, 1990.

Taylor, Timothy. *The Prehistory of Sex: Four Million Years of Human Sexual Culture.* New York: Bantam, 1996.

Tuleja, Tad. *Curious Customs: The Stories Behind 296 Popular American Rituals.* New York: Harmony, 1987.

Walker, Barbara G. *The Women's Encyclopedia of Myths and Secrets.* New York: Harper & Row, 1983.

Walker, Morton. *Foods for Fabulous Sex: Natural Sexual Nutrients to Trigger Passion, Heighten Response, Improve Performance & Overcome Dysfunction.* McKinney, Texas: Magni Group, 1992.

Wallace, Irving. *The Nymphoid and Other Maniacs: The Lives, the Loves and the Sexual Adventures of Some Scandalous and Liberated Ladies.* New York: Simon and Schuster, 1971.

Watson, Cynthia Mervis. *Love Potions: A Guide to Aphrodisiacs and Sexual Pleasures.* New York: Tarcher/Putnam, 1971.

Welch, Leslee. *Sex Facts: A Handbook for the Carnally Curious.* New York: Carol Publishing, 1992.

Wildwood, Chrissie. *Erotic Aromatherapy: Essential Oils for Lovers.* New York: Sterling, 1994.

Worwood, Valerie Ann. *Scents & Scentuality: Aromatherapy & Essential Oils for Romance, Love and Sex.* Novato, Calif.: New World Library, 1999.

Zacks, Richard. *History Laid Bare: Lover Perversity from the Ancient Etruscans to Warren G. Harding.* New York: HarperCollins, 1994.

Zilbergeld, Bernie. *Male Sexuality.* New York: Bantam, 1978.

Zilbergeld, Bernie. *The New Male Sexuality: The Truth About Men, Sex and Pleasure.* Revised Edition. New York: Bantam, 1999.

Zimmerman, Jack and Jacquelyn McCandless. *Flesh and Spirit: The Mystery of the Intimate Relationship.* Las Vegas: Bramble Books, 1998.

Index

A

AARP/*Modern Maturity* Sexuality
    Study, 264
Acknowledgment, 55
Active listening, 72
AFE (anterior fornix erotic) zone
    orgasms, 186
Age, 21–22, 264
Alabama banning of sex toys, 262
Alcohol consumption, 96
Alphabet letters, writing with tongue
    in oral sex, 180
Altoid mints, 235
American Academy of Pediatrics
    (AAP) Committee on the
    Fetus and Newborn, 263–
    264
American Gigolo (film), 223
Anal beads, 238–239
Anal orgasms:
    female, 187
    male, 189

*Anal Pleasure & Health; A Guide for
    Men and Women* (Morin),
    190
Anal sex:
    books on, 190
    and cleanliness, 191
    double penetration of anus and
        vagina, 156
    interest in, reasons for, 253–254
    lubricants for, 191, 254
    and men, 155–156, 253
    myths about, 190
    and relaxation, 191
Anal toys, 155–156, 238–239
Anand, Margot, 149
Anger, 19, 70–71
Anus:
    and Contacting Three Points of
        Pleasure technique, 206
    and Deer Exercise, 209–210
    and male superior intercourse
        position, 194
    See also Anal sex

Aphrodisiacal scents, 147
Appearance, modifying for lover, 18
Appreciation, culture of, 32–34
Argentina, fantasy thinking in, 265
Arguing:
    and attitude, 70–71
    fair fighting, 71–73
Aromatherapy, 147
Arousal:
    women's signs of, 204
    See also Turn-ons
Artichokes, as aphrodisiac, 146
"Art of Exotic Dancing for Everyday
        Women, The" (video), 227
Assumptions, 73
Attention, 55–58, 142
Attitude, 1–49
Avlimil, 17

B

Baby-making sex, 129–132
Back massage, 159
Baker, Chet, 149
Bakos, Susan Crane, 212
Basket Weave hand maneuver,
        171–172
Bath, sex in, 141
Beads, anal, 238–239
Bedroom:
    mirrors in, 157–158
    as sanctuary, 151–152
Bed sheets, 152
Beginner role, 32
Behavior, 51–104
Being-in-love sex vs. falling-in-love
        sex, 1–2
Bend Over Boyfriend video series,
        155, 253
Berries and cream, as aphrodisiac, 146
Best American Erotica, The (Bright),
        143

Best Women's Erotica (Scheiner), 143
Better Than Sex intercourse position,
        201, 202
Birth control, 267–269
Birth control pills, 267
Black, Joel, 212
Blaming, 72
Blended orgasms:
    female, 188
    male, 189
Blindfolded sex, 129
Blue, Violet, 143–145
Body:
    demonstrating love for, 110
    encouraging lover to take care of,
        96
    his body as turn-on for you,
        154–155
    hot spots, 111–112
    loving, 29
    relishing how it makes your lover
        feel, 14–15
    taking care of, 95–96
    turn-on show-and-tell, 112–113
    using his body for your sexual
        pleasure, 122
Body paint, latex, 158
Bondage, 235
Books:
    on anal sex, 190
    erotic, exploring, 143–144
    expanding sexual library, 127
Bored Housewife and Cabana Boy
        fantasy, 223
Bossa Nova (album), 149
Brandy, as aphrodisiac, 146
Breast orgasms, 187
Breasts, and sex in shower, 141
Breath, 73, 97
Breathing techniques:
    basic, 205
    harmonic, 206, 207

Brick, Peggy, 264
Bright, Susie, 143
Britton, Bryce, 213
Brushing hair, 159–160
Bull Durham fantasy, 228
Bungee Sex, 123
Butt plugs, 239

C

Cabana Boy and Bored Housewife
    fantasy, 223
Cabello, Francisco Santa Maria, 256
Cake, as aphrodisiac, 146
Calm before the storm, 14
Cervical caps, 268
Cervical orgasms:
    description of, 185
    and male superior intercourse
        position, 194–196
Chang, Stephen, 209
Chastity belts, modern versions of,
    266
Chemistry, 39–40
Cherishing qualities of lover, 11
Chia, Mantak, 211
Children:
    educating about sex, 255
    infants and skin eroticism, 263
    keeping out of your bed, 83
    smoking and teenage sex, 264
Children-in-the-house sex, 138–139
Chile, fantasy thinking in, 265
Chocolate, as aphrodisiac, 146
Choy, Dominic, 265
Circumcision, 263–265
Cleanliness. *See* Hygiene
Clitoral orgasms, 185
    in blended/fusion orgasm, 188
    and intercourse positions:
        male superior, 194–196
        sitting/kneeling, 201, 202

Clitoris:
    and intercourse positions:
        male superior, 195, 196
        side by side, 197
        sitting/kneeling, 201, 202
    knowledge about, 153
    oral stimulation of:
        alternating broad and pointy
            strokes, 174–175
        avoidance of flicking, 178
        guidance from woman,
            178–179
        kissing, 177–178
        Kivin Method, 175–177
        positions, 173–174
        and sensitivity, 173–175
        training with Lifesavers, 180
        using nose, 175
        using pillows, 179–180
        using underside of tongue, 179
        varying speed and tongue pres-
            sure, 174
        writing alphabet letters with
            tongue, 180
    stimulation by hand:
        It Takes Three maneuver,
            168–170
        Y–Knot maneuver, 170–171
    stimulation with penis, 153
    and Tantric sex:
        Contacting Three Points of
            Pleasure technique, 206
        Uniting the Energy Poles tech-
            nique, 207
Closeness, emotional, 13
Clothing:
    attention to, 39
    and foreplay, 113–114, 116
    undergarments, 102
    well–maintained and clean, 96
Cock rings, 237–238
Code-speak, 106–107

Coitus cloths, 162

Coltrane, John, 149

Coltrane for Lovers (album), 149

Come Away with Me (album), 149

Comfort sex, 129

Comfort zones, challenging, 48

Commitment:
constant awareness of, 44–45
and fair fighting, 73

Common cold, sex and prevention of, 267

Communication, 67
and acting quickly to spot and solve problems, 58–59
asking for something, 74
attitude and arguing, 70–71
code-speak, 106–107
critiquing specific techniques, 118
fair fighting, 71–73
about faked orgasms, 245–246
about fantasies, 218–219, 247
following through on promises, 99–100
of hot spots, 111–112
and intellectual connection, 10–11
of irresistibility, 52, 53
listening. *See* Listening
making each other laugh, 89
about money, 76
and orgasms, 5
phone sex, 225
praising specific techniques, 117
and privacy, 62–63, 65–66
and reinforcement of the relationship foundation, 30
of sexual wants and desires, 61–62
standing up for your rights, 12–13
and support and respect for personal endeavors, 77–78
taking pulse of relationship on ongoing basis, 53–55

talking dirty, 15, 140, 228–229
telephone calls as foreplay, 115, 116
and treating lover as special, 51–52
turning complaints into requests, 86–87
voicing compliments, 99

Compact Massager, 234

Comparisons, avoiding, 63–64

Compartmentalizing, 47

Complacency, 28, 54

Complaints:
gentleness in airing, 19
listening to, 18–19
and relationship "tune-ups," 48
turning into requests, 86–88

Compliments, voicing, 99

Compound single orgasms, 212

Compromise, 25, 67–68

Condoms:
female, 267–268
male, 230–231

Connectedness:
and kissing, 121
as turn-on, 109–111
when apart, 119–120

Conrad, Laurie, 237

Contacting Three Points of Pleasure technique, 206

Contemporary Sexuality, 262, 264–266

Costner, Kevin, 228

Couples therapists, "tune-ups" with, 47–48

Courting spirit, 38–39

C points, 175, 176

Criticisms, turning into requests, 72

Critiquing specific techniques, 118

Crying, 22–23

Cuddling, 101

Curtis, Jamie Lee, 227

D

"Daddy, I've Been Bad" fantasy,
   225–226
Dancing:
   erotic, 227
   as foreplay, 116–117
Davis, Geena, 223
Deer Exercise, 209–210
Deluxe (album), 149
Deluxe Massager, 234
Demands, elimination of, 72
Dental hygiene, 97
Depo-Provera, 268
Desires, communication of, 61–62
Diaphragms, 268
Diet, 95
Dignity, 66
Dildos, 236, 240
Dining:
   feeding each other, 145
   lightly, 118
   reinventing, 92–93
   together, 92
Diplomacy, 66–67
Disciplining fantasy, 225–226
Discretion, 62–63
Doctor Dan and Nurse Nancy
      fantasy, 226–227
Domination/submission fantasy,
   220
Downtime, for partner, 102–103
Dressing, 116
Dress-up fantasy, 222–223
Dry orgasms, 211

E

Ear hairs, 97
Eating. *See* Dining
Edible body paint, 158
Educating children about sex, 255

Ejaculation:
   female, 256
   male, 189
   delaying, 205, 208–210
   and multiple orgasms, 210–211
Embarrassing your lover, avoidance
   of, 65–66
Emission phase of ejaculation, 211
Emotional health, 98
Emotional safety, 85–86
Emotional synergy, 14–15
Emotions:
   and closeness, 13
   crying, 22–23
   effect of negative feelings on sex
      life, 46–47
   touching emotional pulse of part-
      ner, 23–24
Enhancers. *See* Toys
Enzyte, 16
Erections, 251
   morning, 139
   and sex in shower, 141
   and Viagra, 260–261
Erotic books, 143–144
Erotic dancing fantasy, 227
Erotic films, 144–145, 259
Essure, 269
Exercise, 95
Exercises:
   Deer, 209–210
   hip rolls, 214–215
   Kegel, 212–213
   Kegelcisor, 213, 214
   Vaginal Weight Lifting Egg,
      213–214
   washcloth trick, 210
Exhibitionistic/voyeuristic fantasy,
   221
Exotic dancing fantasy, 227
Expectations:
   enlarging, 41–42

Expectations (*cont.*)
minimizing impact of mediaized
messages, 42
Explorer behavior, 60–61
Expulsion phase of ejaculation, 211
Eyes of Desire (film), 145

F

Fair fighting, 71–73
Faked orgasms, 243–246
Falling-in-love sex vs. being-in-love
sex, 1–2
Family:
nurturing values related to,
35–36
support from, 89–90
Fantasies, 217–241
Bored Housewife and Cabana
Boy, 223
Bull Durham, 228
communication about, 218–219,
247
creating, 229–230
"Daddy, I've Been Bad,"
225–226
domination/submission, 220
dress-up, 222–223
erotic dancing, 227
feelings behind, 219
vs. fetishes, 248
guilt about, 247
From Here to Eternity, 227–228
Innocent Schoolgirl, 226
introducing into relationship,
248–249
ménage à trois, 221–222
Nurse Nancy and Doctor Dan,
226–227
Officer and the Gentlewoman, The
224–225

and permission, 3
to assume roles, 220
to discuss, 218
phone sex, 225
Prostitute and the Gentleman,
223–224
readiness for sharing, 17–18
swinging, 222
talking dirty, 228–229
toys, 15–16, 230–241
Alabama banning of, 262
anal, 155–156, 238–239
bondage, 235
cock rings, 237–238
desire to use, meaning of, 254
dildos, 236, 240
harnesses, 239
and interference with sex life, 258
lubricants for, 230–231
openness to, 15–16
pearl necklace, 240–241
and permission, 3
PVC molded, 236–238
shaft sleeves, 237
sources of, 258, 271–282
that vary the senses, 235
untested, potentially harmful
products, 16–17
vibrators, 231–234, 257
voyeuristic/exhibitionistic, 221
worldwide statistics on, 265–266
Fantasy orgasms:
female, 188
male, 189
Fathering Magazine, 266
Feeding each other, 145
Femglide, 231
Femininity, 7–8
Femme Line of vibrators, 234
Feng shui, 84
Fetishes, 248

Fighting fairly, 71–73
Films:
    erotic, 144–145, 259
    horror, 123–124
Finger foods, as aphrodisiac, 146
Fingers, using during oral sex,
        179–180
First-thing-in-the-morning sex, 139
Fisher, Helen, 1–2
Flirting at parties, 117
Food:
    aphrodisiacal, 146
    feeding each other, 145
    -sex connection, 92
    See also Dining
Foreplay, 113–117
    and baby-making sex, 132
    and clothing, 113–114, 116
    dancing as, 116–117
    flirting at parties, 117
    lingering over, 113, 132
    and relaxation, 114
    and sock drawer, 115
    telephone calls as, 115, 116
    and undressing, 116
Forgiveness:
    of lover's human frailties, 46
    maintaining attitude of, 103
    of one's own physical qualities,
        45–46
Foundation of relationship, reinforc-
        ing, 29–30
Frenulum stimulation, 184–185
Frequency of sex, 13–14, 255
Frequent sex, health benefits of, 28
Friends, support from, 89–90
From Here to Eternity fantasy,
        227–228
FSD-Alerting.org, 261
Fun, sex as, 163
Fusion orgasms, 188

G

Gaye, Marvin, 149
Gender identity teams, 266
Gender-role fantasy, 222–223
Genital hygiene, 97–98
Gentleman and Prostitute fantasy,
        223–224
Gentlemanly behavior, 4–5
Gentlewoman and the Officer
        fantasy, 224–225
Gere, Richard, 223
Gilberto, Joao, 149
Giving, gift of, 20
Gottman, John, 25
Graduate, The (film), 223
Grafenberg, Ernst, 252
Grievances. *See* Complaints
Grooming, 96–97
Groundhog Day (film), 56
G spot:
    and intercourse positions:
        female superior, 192
        male superior, 195, 196
        rear entry, 198–199
        side by side, 197–198
        sitting/kneeling, 201, 202
    locating, 154
    and Tantric sex:
        Contacting Three Points of
            Pleasure technique, 206
        Kneeling at the Gate of Plea-
            sure technique, 207
        Uniting the Energy Poles tech-
            nique, 206–207
G spot orgasms, 186, 252–253

H

Hair:
    brushing and washing, 159–160

Hair (*cont.*)
  nose and ear, 97
  pubic, 97
Haircuts, 96
Hand maneuvers, 86
  Basket Weave, 171–172
  It Takes Three, 168–170
  Ode to Bryan, 166–168
  Y-Knot, 170–171
Harlequin Enterprises, 265
Harmonic breathing, 206, 207
Harnesses, 239
Hart, Veronica, 144, 145
Health:
  benefits of frequent sex, 28
  emotional, 98
  mental, 98
Healthy Immunity, 267
Hearing, sense of, 149
Heart to Heart Loving technique,
      207–208
Her Turn, 17
Hide-and-seek sex, 128
Hip rolls, 214–215
Hitachi Magic Wand, 233
Honesty:
  about lover's human frailties, 46
  about one's own physical qualities,
      45–46
Honey, as aphrodisiac, 146
Horror films, 123–124
Hotel sex, 93
How to Make Love All Night
      (Keesling), 211
HPV (human papilloma virus),
      265
Hug and Run, 82
Hugging, 84–85, 100–101
Human frailties of lover, honesty and
      forgiveness about, 46
Humor, 89

Hygiene, 97
  and anal sex, 191
  awareness of, 73

I

Immunoglobulin, 267
Infants and skin eroticism, 263
Initiation of sex, by women, 124,
      156
Inner voice, listening to, 79–80
Innocent Schoolgirl fantasy, 226
Instant gratification, 75
Intellectual connection, 10–11
Intercourse, 2–3
  and female orgasms, 246
  new idea sources, 257
  positions, 191–204
    female superior, 192–194
    male superior, 194–196
    rear entry, 198–200
    side by side, 196–198
    sitting/kneeling, 200–202
    standing, 203–204
    sucking penis into vagina, 214
Intersex condition, 266
ISNA (Intersex Society of North
      America), 266
It Takes Three hand maneuver,
      168–170
IUDs, 268
"I Want You" (song), 149

J

Japan, fantasy thinking in, 265–266
Japanese meditation box, 160
Jaye-Brandt, Jackie, 72–73
Jealousy, 68–69
"Je ne sais quoi" ("I just can't explain
      it"), 39–40

Jones, Norah, 149
Juette, Astrid, 262

𝒦

Kama Sutra, 144
Kaschak, Ellyn, 261
Keesling, Barbara, 211
Kegelcisor, 213, 214
Kegel exercises, 212–213
Kerr, Deborah, 227–228
Kinison, Sam, 55, 180
Kissing:
    frequency, 121
    and oral sex, 177–178
    preferences, 120
Kivin Method, 175–177
Kneeling at the Gate of Pleasure
        technique, 207
Kneeling intercourse position,
        200–202
K points, 175, 176

𝓛

Labels, 72
Lancaster, Burt, 227–228
Lane, Diane, 249
Language, explicit, 15, 140, 228–229
Late-afternoon sex, 140
Latex body paint, 158
Laughter, 89
Learning about sex:
    openness to, 3
    and permission, 3
Leather clothing, 263
Leslie, John, 144–145
Liberated Orgasm (Otto), 187
Library, sexual, 127, 143–144
Lifesavers, training for oral sex with,
        180

Lifestyle choice, lovemaking as, 44
Lingering over foreplay, 113, 132
Liqueur, as aphrodisiac, 146
Liquid Silk, 231
Listening:
    active, 72
    as attention, 56
    to complaints, 18–19
    to inner voice, 79–80
Living organism, relationship as,
        76–77
Locations for sex:
    bath, 141
    bedroom as sanctuary, 151–152
    and children-in-the-house sex,
        138–139
    shower, 140–141
    steamroom, 141–142
    unexpected, 124–125
    unfamiliar, 156–157
Lollypops, as aphrodisiac, 146
Love-life response sheet, 112
Lovemaking styles, 127–140
    Baby-making, 129–132
    blindfolded, 129
    children-in-the-house, 138–139
    first-thing-in-the-morning, 139
    hide-and-seek, 128
    late-afternoon, 140
    middle-of–the-night, 137–138
    pleasures of comfort, 129
    pregnancy positions, 132–137
    silence-is-golden, 128
Love Muscle, The (Britton), 213
Love's Passion (film), 145
Love vs. lust, 11–12
Lubricants:
    for anal sex, 191, 254
    basic information on, 161–162
    for toys, 230–231
Lunelle, 268

Lust:
  vs. love, 11–12
  and triumvirate of the body, 29

M

MacDowell, Andie, 56
Male superior intercourse position,
  194–196
Mangoes, as aphrodisiac, 146
Manners, 4–5, 26–27, 39, 162
Martinez, Olivier, 249
Masculinity, 7–8
Massage:
  back, 159
  scalp, 159
Masturbation, 259–260
Maximus, 231
Maxwell Urban Suite, 149
McClintock, Martha, 262
Media, 42, 64, 244
Meditation, 95, 206
Meditation box, Japanese, 160
Memories, attention to, 88–89
Ménage à trois, 221–222
Men's Health magazine, 94
Menstrual cycles and pheromones,
  262
Mental health, 98
Mess, not worrying about, 127
Middle-of-the-night sex, 137–138
Midnite Fire, 231
Milbank Quarterly, The, 264
Mirrors, 157–158
Mistakes, learning from, 59–60
Money:
  communicating about, 76
  nurturing values related to,
  37–38
Mood, sex despite, 142–143
Morin, Jack, 190
Morning erections, 139

Mouth orgasms:
  female, 187
  male, 189
Muir, Caroline, 206, 208
Muir, Charles, 206, 208
Multi-Orgasmic Male, The (Chia),
  211
Multiple orgasms:
  female, 211–212
  male, 210–211
Multi-Satisfier, 234
Murray, Bill, 56
Music, 149
Mutuality, spirit of, 24–25
Mutual respect, 19–20

N

Nails, 97
Negative energy, focusing on,
  103
Negative feelings, effect on sex life,
  46–47
Negotiating skills, 66–67
*New England Journal of Medicine,
  The,* 265
New Male Sexuality, The (Zilber-
  geld), 3
*New View of Women's Sexual Prob-
  lems, A* (Tiefer and Kaschak),
  261
New York Times, The, 264
Nipple orgasms:
  female, 187
  male, 189
Nipple vibrators, 233
Nonoxynol-9, 162
Nose, using in oral sex, 175
Nose hairs, 97
Nurse Nancy and Doctor Dan fantasy,
  226–227
Nuvaring, 268

O

Ode to Bryan hand maneuver,
    166–168
Officer and the Gentlewoman
    fantasy, 224–225
Oils, massage, 159
One Size Fits All (film), 145
Openness:
    to enhancers, 15–16
    to learning about sex, 3
    to other's viewpoint, 25
Oral sex:
    after marriage or commitment,
        6–7
    on men, 180–185
        eye contact, 180
        frenulum stimulation, 184–185
        frequency of, 251–252
        Ring and Seal maneuver,
            181–183
        swallowing, 259
        and taste of semen, 250–251
        testicles, 183–184
        women's attitude towards, 6
    on women, 173–180
        alternating broad and pointy
            strokes, 174–175
        avoidance of flicking, 178
        guidance from woman,
            178–179
        kissing, 177–178
        Kivin Method, 175–177
        positions, 173–174
        sensitivity of clitoris, 173–175
        and taste of secretions, 250–251
        training with Lifesavers, 180
        using nose, 175
        using pillows, 179–180
        using underside of tongue, 179
        varying speed and tongue pres-
            sure, 174

writing alphabet letters with
    tongue, 180
Orgasms:
    and breathing, 205
    delaying, 205, 208–210
    faked, 243–246
    female:
        AFE (anterior fornix erotic)
            zone, 186
        anal, 187
        blended/fusion, 188
        breast/nipple, 187
        cervical, 185, 195
        clitoral, 185, 195
        fantasy, 188
        G spot, 186, 252–253
        intention to elicit, 5
        and intercourse, 195, 246
        mouth, 187
        multiple, 211–212
        removing as goal, 31
        statistics about, 261
        urethral, 186, 188–189, 195
        vaginal, 185
        zone, 188
    male:
        multiple, 210–211
        types of, 189
        and permission, 3
Ortho Evra, 268–269
Otto, Herbert A., 187
Outings, 94
Oxytocin, 125
Oysters, as aphrodisiac, 146

P

Paint, body, 158
Paraurethral glands, 256
Parties:
    flirting at, 117
    having sex during, 157

Passion, sex as, 43

Patience, 74

PC (pubococcygeus) muscle,
     209–215
  and Deer Exercise, 209–210
  and female orgasms, 245
  and hip rolls, 214–215
  and Kegelcisor, 213, 214
  and Kegel exercises, 212–213
  and male multi-orgasms, 211
  and Vaginal Weight Lifting Egg,
     213–214
  and washcloth trick, 210

Pearl necklace, as toy, 240–241

Pearsall, Paul, 28

Pelvic/hypogastric nerve system, 185,
     188, 252

Penile orgasms, 189

Penis
  and circumcision, 263–265
  erections, 251
     morning, 139
     and sex in shower, 141
     and Viagra, 260–261
  and hand maneuvers:
     Basket Weave, 171–172
     Ode to Bryan hand maneuver,
       166–168
  and intercourse positions:
     female superior, 192
     rear entry, 199
  oral stimulation of: See Oral
  sex; on men stimulating clitoris
     with, 153
  studying reactions to stimulation
     of, 152–153
  sucking into vagina, 214
  and washcloth trick, 210

Performance, 43

Perineum, 176, 179

Permission:
  to assume roles in fantasies, 220

  to discuss fantasies, 218
  and toys, 3

Personal boundaries, 13

Personal disclosure, 62–63

Personal endeavors, support and
     respect for, 77–78

Pheromones, 262

Phone sex, 225

Photographs, 110

Physical qualities, and honesty and
     self-forgiveness, 45–46

Pink Elephant, 236–237

Pitt, Brad, 223

Planning:
  outings, 94
  sex, 94–95
  sexual scenarios, 122–123
  trips, 93

Playbook of tips and techniques,
     105–163

"Playing doctor," grownup version
     of, 226–227

Pocket-Rocket vibrator, 232

Portishead, 149

Praise, 55, 117

Pregnancy sex, 132–137, 200, 201

Preven kits, 268

Pride, lover's, 25–26

Privacy, 62–63, 65–66, 162

Private time, 91

Problem solving:
  accepting limitations on, 30–31
  acting quickly, 58–59
  and fair fighting, 72

Promises, following through on,
     99–100

Prostate, stimulation of, 155, 188,
     239

Prostate orgasms, 189

Prostitute and the Gentleman fantasy,
     223–224

Pubic hair, 97

Pudendal nerve system, 252
Pushing each other's buttons, 69
PVC molded toys, 236–238

Q

Qualities of lover, cherishing, 11

R

Rabbit Pearl vibrator, 232
Reagan, Nancy, 26
Reality female condom, 267–268
Rear entry intercourse position,
    198–200
Receiving sexually, 20–21
Refuge, relationship as, 9–10
Reggae, 149
Rejuvenation, and sex, 28–29
Rekindling sex life, 260
Relaxation:
    and anal sex, 191
    brushing and washing hair,
        159–160
    and foreplay, 114
    giving partner downtime,
        102–103
    meditation, 95
    spending time alone, 91
    See also Massage
Requests:
    code-speak, 106–107
    framing, 74
    turning complaints into, 86–88
Resolution-oriented fighting, 72
Respect:
    mutual, 19–20
    for personal endeavors, 77–78
Response sheet, love-life, 112
Responsibility, and fair fighting, 72
Reward, sex as, 43
Right, insistence on being, 24–25

Rights, standing up for, 12–13
Rimming, 187
Ring and Seal maneuver, 181–183
Romancing, 64–65
Roman Orgy Love Oil, 159
Rose Petals technique, 187
Royalle, Candida, 144, 145, 234

S

Sade, 149
Safety, emotional, 85–86
Sand, Japanese meditation box of,
    160
Sarandon, Susan, 228
Sarcasm, 66, 72
Scalp massage, 159
Scents:
    aphrodisiacal, 147
    natural, 154, 250
Scheiner, Marcy, 143
Schoolgirl fantasy, 226
Schwarzenegger, Arnold, 227
Seasonal Sex game, 40
Secrets of the Super Young (Weeks),
    28
Self-forgiveness of physical qualities,
    45–46
Semen:
    leaving inside, 125–126
    production of, 209
    swallowing, 259
    taste of, 250–251
Seniors and sex, 22, 264
Sensual atmosphere in home, 84
Sensuality, expanding, 146–151
    hearing, 149
    smell, 147, 148
    taste, 151
    touch, 150–151
    visual, 148–149
Sensura, 231

Sequential multiple orgasms, 212

Serial multiple orgasms, 212

Sex:

  as priority, 22

  as privilege not work, 26

  rushing into, 74–75

Sex Grease, 231

Sex over 50 (Black and Bakos), 212

Sexual comfort zones, challenging, 48

Sexual cues, 106

Sexual dysfunction, 261

Sexual frequency. *See* Frequency of sex

Sexual history, 8

Sexual inspiration, 118–119

Sexual library, 127

Sexual moments and memories, attention to, 88

Sexual scenarios, planning, 122–123

Shaft sleeves, 237

Shane, 144, 145

Shane's World videos, 145

Shaving:

  her, 161

  him, 160–161

Sheets, 152

Shore, Dinah, 22–23

Show-and-tell of turn-ons, 112–113

Shower, sex in, 140–141

Shunga, 148

Side-by-side intercourse position, 196–198

Sight, sense of, 148–149

Silence-is-golden lovemaking style, 128

Silk panties, 174

Sitting intercourse position, 200–202

Skin, 80

Skin eroticism, roots of, 263

Skinny-dipping, 142

"Sky Dancing Tantra: A Call to Bliss" (song), 149

Sleep, adequate, 95

Slippery Stuff, 141, 231

Smell, sense of, 147, 148

Smoking:

  and taste of genital secretions, 251

  and teenage sex, 264

Sock drawer, 115

Songs for Lovers (album), 149

South America, fantasy thinking in, 265

Space, giving, 78

Spanking, 158, 225, 226

Spark, lack of, 260

Spermicides, vaginal, 268

Sphincters, anal, 191, 254

Spiritual life, nurturing values related to, 35–36

Spontaneous actions, 23

Spooning, 137, 138

Sportsheets, 235

Standing intercourse position, 203–204

Steamroom, sex in, 141–142

Stonewalling, 25

Stories, allowing partner to take credit for, 90

Stress, fighting for relationship in times of, 78–79

Style differences, 45

Submission/domination fantasy, 220

Superimmunity (Pearsall), 28

Support:

  from friends and family, 89–90

  for personal endeavors, 77–78

Surprise, 126

Swallowing semen, 259

Sweet Life (Blue), 143–144

Swinging, 222

Swirl, the, 150–151

𝒯

Tactile eroticism, 80–82
Talking dirty, 15, 140, 228–229
Tantra: The Art of Conscious Loving
    (Muir and Muir), 206
Tantric sex, 205–208
    Contacting Three Points of Plea-
        sure technique, 206
    defined, 205–206
    and delaying ejaculation, 205, 208
    Heart to Heart Loving technique,
        207–208
    Kneeling at the Gate of Pleasure
        technique, 207
    Uniting the Energy Poles tech-
        nique, 206–207
Tao of Sexology, The (Chang), 209
Taormino, Tristan, 190
Taste:
    of female ejaculate, 256
    of semen, 250–251
    sense of, 151
    of vaginal secretions, 250–251
Taylor, Tina, 144
Teenage sex and smoking, 264
Telephone calls:
    and connectedness when apart, 119
    as foreplay, 115, 116
    phone sex, 225
Television:
    as distraction, 83
    as preparation for sex, 123–124
Tensions, effect on sex life, 46–47
Ten Ways Women Can Be Stimu-
    lated for Orgasm, 165
Testicles:
    and Deer Exercise, 209
    and male superior intercourse
        position, 194, 195
    and oral sex, 183–184
    and sex in shower, 141

Thelma and Louise (film), 223
Tiefer, Leonore, 261
Timetable for sex, avoidance of,
    40–41
Tina Tyler's Going Down (film), 145
Today Sponge, 269
Tongue:
    and oral sex on men: in Ring and
        Seal maneuver, 182
    and oral sex on women:
        and anal orgasms, 187
        speed and pressure, 174
        using underside of, 174
        writing alphabet letters with, 180
Tongue Joy vibrator, 233–234
Touching, 150–151
    cuddling, 101
    hugging, 84–85, 100–101
    maintaining connection, 100
    skills, 80–82
    the Swirl, 150–151
Toys, 15–16, 230–241
    Alabama banning of, 262
    anal, 155–156, 238–239
    bondage, 235
    cock rings, 237–238
    desire to use, meaning of, 254
    dildos, 236, 240
    harnesses, 239
    and interference with sex life,
        258
    lubricants for, 230–231
    openness to, 15–16
    pearl necklace, 240–241
    and permission, 3
    PVC molded, 236–238
    shaft sleeves, 237
    sources of, 258, 271–282
    that vary the senses, 235
    untested, potentially harmful
        products, 16–17
    vibrators, 231–234, 257

Traveling, 93
Travel Massager, 234
Trip planning, 93
Trouble, looking for, 101–102
True Lies (film), 227
Trust, 9, 85–86
"Tune-ups," 47–48
Turn-offs:
    for men, 111
    for women, 108–109
Turn-ons:
    hot spots, 111–112
    love-life response sheet, 112
    scent, 154
    show–and–tell, 112–113
    for women, 106
        connectedness, 109–111
        demonstrating love for body,
            110
        knowledge of, 107–108
        man's body, 154–155
Tyler, Tina, 145

U

*Ultimate Guide to Adult Videos, The:
    How to Watch Adult Videos
    and Make Your Sex Life Sizzle*
    (Blue), 144
*Ultimate Guide to Anal Sex for
    Women* (Taormino), 190
Ultimate Massager, 234
Undergarments, 102
Undressing, and foreplay, 116
Unexpected locations, sex in,
    124–125
Unexpected sexual approaches,
    126
Unfaithful (film), 249
Unfamiliar locations, sex in,
    156–157

Uniqueness, 63–64
Uniting the Energy Poles technique,
    206–207
Urethral (U–spot) orgasms, 186,
    188–189, 194–196

V

Vagina:
    and It Takes Three hand maneu-
        ver, 168–170
    and lubricants, 231
    oral stimulation of. *See* Oral sex:
        on women
    sucking penis into, 214
Vaginal orgasms, 185
    in blended/fusion orgasm, 188
    and male superior intercourse
        position, 194–196
Vaginal spermicides, 268
Vaginal Weight Lifting Egg,
    213–214
Valentine's Day, 49
Values in common, nurturing,
    34–38
    family, 34–35
    money, 37–38
    spiritual life, 35–36
    work, 36–37
Verbal cueing, 106
Very Private, 231
ViaCream, 16
Viagra, 260–261
Vibrators, 231–234, 257
Videos, 144–145
Video Voyeur, 240
Viewpoint, openness to, 25
Virtual reality sex, 265
Visual, sense of, 148–149
Vitamin depletion, and birth control
    pills, 267

Vomeronasal organs (VNO), 262
Voyeuristic/exhibitionistic fantasy, 221
Voyeur series (Leslie), 144–145
Vulnerability, 8–9

W

Washcloths, bedside, 162
Washcloth trick, 210
Washing hair, 159–160
Water-based lubricants, 161, 231, 254
Weeks, David, 28
Whipple, Beverly, 186, 252
White Lightning (film), 145
Wilder, Esther, 264

Work:
 downtime on return from, 102–103
 nurturing values related to, 36–37

Y

Yeast infections, 231, 250
Y–Knot hand maneuver, 170–171
Yoga, 95

Z

Zilbergeld, Bernie, 3, 21–22
Zone orgasms:
 female, 188
 male, 189